The International Behavioural and Social Sciences Library

STUDIES OF TROUBLESOME CHILDREN

TAVISTOCK

The International Behavioural and Social Sciences Library

CHILD DEVELOPMENT
In 9 Volumes

STUDIES OF TROUBLESOME CHILDREN

D H STOTT

Routledge
Taylor & Francis Group
LONDON AND NEW YORK

First published in 1966 by
Tavistock Publications Limited

Published in 2001 by
Routledge
2 Park Square, Milton Park, Abingdon, Oxfordshire OX14 4RN
711 Third Avenue, New York, NY 10017

First issued in paperback 2014

Routledge is an imprint of the Taylor & Francis Group, an informa company

British Library Cataloguing in Publication Data
A CIP catalogue record for this book
is available from the British Library

Studies of Troublesome Children

Child Development: 9 Volumes

The International Behavioural and Social Sciences Library
112 Volumes

ISBN 978-0-415-26400-6 (hbk)
ISBN 978-0-415-75357-9 (pbk)

Studies of Troublesome Children

D. H. STOTT M.A., Ph.D.

Professor and Head of the Department of Psychology
University of Guelph, Ontario

Formerly Lecturer in Psychology
University of Glasgow

TAVISTOCK PUBLICATIONS

HUMANITIES PRESS

First published in Great Britain in 1966
by Tavistock Publications Ltd

First published in the United States of America in 1966
by Humanities Press Inc.

Library of Congress Catalog Card Number 66–15541
A version of the first part of this book
was published in 1964 as a
Convocation Lecture of the National Children's Home
under the title of
'Thirty-three Troublesome Children'

Contents

The Convocation Lectureship of the National Children's Home

At the Convocation of 1945 the workers of the National Children's Home decided to institute a CONVOCATION LECTURESHIP and for this purpose to invite to the Annual Convocation a distinguished exponent of some aspect of child-welfare practice.

It was further agreed that the series of Convocation Lectures thus constituted should be published and circulated as widely as possible as a timely contribution towards the solution of some of the most important and pressing problems of child care.

The former lectures in this series are:

1946 'The Purpose of the Family', by Sir J. C. Spence, M.D., F.R.C.P.; Nuffield Professor of Child Health in the University of Durham.

1947 'The Foundations of Health in Childhood', by Norman B. Capon, M.D., F.R.C.P.; Professor of Child Health in the University of Liverpool.

1948 'The Religious Basis of Education', by J. S. Ross, C.B.E., M.A., B.SC.; Principal, Westminster Training College.

1949 'The Substitute Family', by Frances Knight, L.H.D.; Director Emeritus, Methodist Children's Home Society, Children's Village, Detroit, Michigan, U.S.A.

1950 'Children as Citizens', by Margery Fry, J.P., LL.D., D.C.L.

1951 'Abnormalities in Normal Children', by C. W. Valentine, M.A., D.PHIL.; Emeritus Professor of Education in the University of Birmingham.

1952 'The Causes and Treatment of Backwardness', by Sir Cyril Burt, D.SC., HON. LITT.D., HON. LL.D.; Fellow of the British Academy; Honorary Fellow, Jesus College, Oxford; Emeritus Professor of Psychology, University of London; formerly Psychologist to the London County Council.

1953 'The Roots of Parenthood', by John Bowlby, M.D.; Director of Department for Children and Parents, Tavistock Clinic, London.

1954 'I sat where They sat', by Rev. John H. Litten, C.B.E.; formerly Principal, National Children's Home.

1955 'Heredity and Environment in Human Affairs', by L. S. Penrose, M.D., F.R.S.; Galton Professor of Eugenics, University College, London.

1956 'The Changing Child', by Alan Moncrieff, C.B.E., M.D., F.R.C.P., J.P.; Nuffield Professor of Child Health, University of London; Physician, The Hospital for Sick Children, Great Ormond Street, London.

1957 'Progress in Child Care', by Audrey Wilson, M.A.; Principal, Princess Alice College, Sutton Coldfield.

1958 'Physical Maturing and Behaviour at Adolescence', by J. M. Tanner, M.D., D.SC., D.P.M.; Senior Lecturer in Growth and Development, Institute of Child Health, University of London.

1959 'Child of Our Times', by W. D. Wall, M.A., PH.D.; Director of the National Foundation for Educational Research in England and Wales.

1960 'The Concept of Love in Child Care', by T. S. Simey, M.A.; Charles Booth Professor of Social Science, University of Liverpool.

1961 'The Whole Child', by Alex G. Mearns, M.B.A., M.D., B.SC., D.P.H., F.R.S.E.; Senior Lecturer in Social Medicine, University of Glasgow.

1962 'Children not Cases', by Kenneth Brill, O.B.E., LL.B., A.A.P.S.W.; Children's Officer, County of Devon.

1963 'The Religious Needs of Children in Care', by the Rev. H. A. Hamilton, B.A.; formerly Principal, Westhill Training College, Selly Oak; Chairman, Congregational Union of England and Wales, 1961–62.

Acknowledgements

The writer wishes to place on record his appreciation of the facilities granted to him by the Corporation of Glasgow Education Committee for the conduct of the study reported in Part I, and his gratitude to the School Welfare Officers for their ever-patient cooperation.

He has also to acknowledge his indebtedness to the National Association of Education Welfare Officers who – thanks to the organizing talents of their secretary, Mr A. R. Millington – provided the data for the study of truants which is the subject of Part II.

Thanks are due to the following for permission to quote from the sources listed below: Miss Margaret Procter, in respect of her article 'Tutorial classes'; the editor of *The Times Educational Supplement*, in respect of the article by J. B. Mays that appeared in the issue of 24 November 1961; the Editor of the *Journal of Psychosomatic Research*, in respect of 'Some psychosomatic aspects of casualty in reproduction' by D. H. Stott, published in Volume 3, Number 1, 1959; E. & S. Livingstone Limited, Edinburgh, in respect of *The growth and development of the prematurely born infant by* C. M. Drillien.

Introduction

The study reported in Part I of this book was undertaken in 1961, soon after the Delinquency Prediction Instrument was made available. The Corporation of Glasgow Education Committee granted facilities to the writer to carry out a small experiment in the detection and prevention of delinquency in cooperation with their School Welfare Officers.

The School Welfare Officers constitute a comparatively small service that is in course of development. So far as the writer knows this service is unique in Britain. Its value for delinquency prevention and for dealing with emotional problems within schools is discussed in a later chapter. At the time that the research was conducted it was composed of twelve qualified social workers, each of whom was based on a single secondary school in a high-delinquency area (one of the schools had a primary department). For the purposes of the investigation that was planned the service offered several advantages. The social workers were members of the school staffs and had daily contact with the teachers in the staff rooms; therefore they were not merely cooperating with the schools but belonged to the same organization. They were recognized as being the means of liaison between the schools and the parents, and their chief duty was to visit the home concerned when a teacher reported that a child showed signs of being neglected or was presenting a disciplinary problem beyond the normal means of correction. However, since they also carried out home visits on routine welfare matters such as the provision of school meals, they were not looked upon by the parents as harbingers of trouble. In many cases they were accepted as friends and guides, and gained insight into the family's situation and difficulties. Thus they were in an admirable position for organizing situational treatment and for coordinating the efforts of other social agencies.

It was decided to focus the inquiry on a complete year's entry into the twelve secondary schools covered by the School Welfare Officer service. The children selected in this way were aged between twelve and thirteen years. The aim was to see whether, by detecting the delinquency prone and treating a proportion of them by family casework methods, the onset of delinquency could be averted.

For each child a teacher marked Yes or No in answer to the six questions of the preliminary sorting procedure of the Delinquency Prediction Instrument.[75]* These questions cover broadly the types of behaviour disturbance most typical of delinquents. For those children for whom three or more adverse answers were given – indicating a strong probability of delinquency proneness – the teachers were asked to complete the full Bristol School Adjustment Guides, from which a delinquency-prediction score was obtained. If this score confirmed the delinquency proneness the case was brought before a conference consisting of the full team of Social Welfare Officers and the writer. The object was to arrive at as thorough a diagnosis as possible of the child's disturbed behaviour and to decide upon a form of situational treatment. In the main this consisted in an attempt to influence the child's family and school environment in order to remove or lessen sources of insecurity or other stress.

It very soon became apparent that no formal experiment would be practicable. First, it was found that a large proportion of the children picked out as delinquency prone had already been before the courts. The test should have been applied two or three years earlier. Second, the Welfare Officers had a general responsibility for all children in need of their guidance so that no control group of disturbed children could be left untreated. Moreover the influence of the Welfare Officers within the schools was pervasive. When one or two of a difficult group are selected for treatment, the situation is altered for others not specifically treated; if teachers learn to regard troublesomeness in one child as a form of behaviour disturbance they are likely to take the same view of other troublesome children and modify their handling of them accordingly. Third, the social workers were concerned about a certain number of other children who were outside the age-group that was being systematically assessed, and expressed a wish to bring them up for consideration in the case conferences. In the event, thirty-three troublesome children were selected as subjects, and their cases are reported in detail in the first part of this volume.

* See Appendix I, p. 185 below.

The attempt to graft a piece of research onto the regular work of the service entailed a further drawback. The depth to which any case could be investigated was limited to what might be of value in dealing with it from a therapeutic point of view. For this reason the conclusions about causation that are drawn from this study must be regarded as tentative, and as pointing rather to the need for more exhaustive research by a team able to devote the requisite time to the collection of more detailed and systematic data.

Nevertheless, the case conferences themselves constituted an experiment in therapeutic method. The procedures used and the lessons learnt from them are detailed in Chapter Six and Appendix IV. As far as the thirty-three cases are concerned, they may be said to offer a fair sample of the kinds of behaviour problem met in a city secondary school serving an inner city neighbourhood. They also raise the question of the resources that would be required for the alleviation of the situation; some tentative proposals on this issue are put forward in Chapter Six.

Questions of individual therapy and of re-educative facilities have to be answered against a background of an understanding of the causes of behaviour disturbance. For long the writer had been dissatisfied with the contemporary assumption – to challenge which must to many seem like heresy – that maladjustment can be explained entirely in terms of the influences acting upon the individual from birth. Among these the most often adduced are defects in the child/parent relationships, especially the warmth of the relationship with the mother. Recently, during a radio discussion of the high suicide rate among students at Oxford and Cambridge, a psychiatrist who was attached to the latter university expressed the view that suicide is the result of emotional deprivation in early childhood. According to this judgement, where the individual concerned has been brought up in his own family, the blame for his suicide is placed squarely on the parents. It has become part of our folklore that delinquency and maladjustment are indications of parental failure. This may often, or usually, be so; but what we have to be sure of, before we confidently explain suicide or other aberrant behaviour along these lines, is that the connection is inevitably a causal one. We need to discover, by the systematic study of instances, whether the relationship between a stressful or depriving family situation and behaviour disturbance in the child always holds. Does *every* child brought up in an adverse situation become maladjusted? And are there ever any patently disturbed children in what – so far as we are able to discover – are stable, loyal, affectionate, well-regulated families?

It is very easy, when we cannot discover any failure of affection or loyalty, to fall back upon the assumption that there must have been some subtle deprivation or lack of warm contact between the child and the mother. But this is not the method of science; once we fill in the gaps in our explanations by assuming what cannot be verified we are methodologically putting the cart before the horse. Instead of questioning our concepts when they do not tally with experience, we would be imagining facts convenient to our hypothesis. In the same way, when we find one disturbed or delinquent child among stable siblings, we are tempted to say in explanation that the situation within the family is different for each sibling. In many cases this is undoubtedly true: we find that one child is rejected and another accepted. But we should go on to ask whether there was something about a particular child in the first place that might have caused him to be rejected. Second, we should proceed to verify that the disturbed child's family situation is significantly different from that of his siblings, and not just suppose it to be so. When one discusses this question with parents in relation to their own children they will almost certainly remark how unlike each other their children are in temperament and personality, and yet they are unaware of having treated them differently. They may of course have done so unconsciously. But to assume that they must have done so once more implies that very small and subtle differences in the human environment can produce striking differences in personality. Again, this cannot be categorically denied; but until it is demonstrated we cannot legitimately build a theory upon it. At the best the hypothesis must be only a tentative one, which will have to give way to another that might explain the facts more comprehensively and in ways that can be verified.

It is a common observation that disturbed children tend to be members of unstable, stressful families. The underlying aim of the research was to re-examine critically, in the light of the thirty-three selected cases, this widespread belief in the relationship between behaviour disturbance and unfavourable family environment and, if it became clear that the influences to which the children in question were exposed in the course of their upbringing fell short of providing a complete explanation of their difficulties, to seek other possible factors. A corollary of the postnatal environmentalist theory would be that the type of behaviour disturbance should tally with the type of deprivation experienced. This formed a secondary aspect of the inquiry.

Part II presents a study of three hundred truants, carried out in cooperation with the Education Welfare Officers' National Association. Various popular conceptions about the type of child who truants were seen to be unfounded. This survey also served to throw light upon a lively current controversy – whether what the middle class sees as deviant behaviour in other subcultural groups is intrinsic maladjustment, or just the accepted behaviour of typical, well-adjusted young people in an inner-urban working-class neighbourhood.

Part III discusses the wider implications of these and related research findings for an understanding of behaviour disturbance.

In recent years there has been a growing volume of evidence that behaviour disturbance is intimately related to other forms of impairment. That which seemed to the writer most cogent is summarized in Chapter Eight. The conclusion drawn is that what may be called a law of multiple congenital impairment is central to the understanding of behaviour disturbance and to clinical diagnosis.

An outline of the writer's typology of maladjustment is given in Chapter Nine. But so that the treatment should not appear unduly dogmatic it takes the form of a description of how he arrived at his concepts and of how he is now inclined to modify the typology upon which the Bristol Social Adjustment Guides are based. From the data of the reported studies a further syndrome, that of inconsequence, crystallized in the writer's mind.

Finally, any theory of abnormal behaviour must be founded upon a general theory of human behaviour and motivation. The writer's is stated briefly in Chapter Ten.

PART I

Thirty-three Troublesome Children

CHAPTER ONE

Children in Stable Families

The Research Procedure

In attempting to elucidate the causal factors underlying behaviour disturbance the writer was led to question the widely accepted view that it can be largely explained in terms of unfavourable environmental influences, particularly the quality of the child–parent relationships. An opportunity arose to test the validity of this view in relation to the sample of troublesome children whose selection has been outlined in the Introduction.

Some means of identifying and classifying depriving family situations was required for this purpose. That adopted was the set of twelve 'patterns' of adverse child–parent relationships arrived at by a study group of Bristol social workers in conjunction with the writer.[56]* The thirty-three children were divided into three groups. One group consisted of fifteen children in whose families one of these adverse patterns was recognizable. Another group contained thirteen cases: in eleven of these, elements of one of the patterns, or some other stressful features, were present, but not at a critical level such as might be held completely to account for the emotional disturbance; in the remaining two instances included in this group the child had been parted from the mother in the pre-school years but brought up in a stable family with a surrogate mother. Finally, there was a group of five apparently stable families which nonetheless contained children who showed disturbance in school.

* The twelve patterns of adverse child–parent relationships are presented in Appendix II, together with the categories of maladjustment that are referred to in this work. Both the adverse family situations and the categories of maladjustment are identified by appropriate capital letters. To avoid possible confusion, the family situations are referred to as *patterns* and the varieties of maladjustment as *types* throughout the text.

This small group presented a theoretical challenge in that they seemed to contradict the contemporary assumption that maladjustment is necessarily related to grossly adverse childhood experience. The children enjoyed the security of stable families and had never been separated from their parents for any appreciable length of time. For this reason they are the first group to be examined, on the principle that the case that does not fit the hypothesis is most likely to provide new insight.

Criteria of Stability

Before the cases are described, two questions have to be asked: first, what constitutes a stable family; and second, in these five families classified as stable, could familial causes of maladjustment have remained undiscovered? To deal first with the latter point: it is unlikely that the School Welfare Officers would have been unaware of grossly deleterious situations. They had routine opportunities for visiting the parents and, operating as they did for a fairly lengthy period within a small neighbourhood, they got to know the local people. No doubt each of these families, like every other, had its phases of stress, but they were contained and dealt with in the family itself. This last statement can probably be taken as a good working definition of a stable family, and thus it provides us with an answer to the first question. If stresses have reached a point where they threaten the unity and continued existence of the family, the mother will hardly be able, or want, to put on a front of having no worries, of having amicable relations with her husband, and so on. Since these were mainly working-class families there were economic stresses, and some of the mothers with large families must have been overburdened. But it speaks for the stability of the parents that even so they were able to provide a secure family life for their children.

The best measure of their success in doing so was that none of the thirty-two siblings showed serious maladjustment. One girl, aged fourteen, was described as harum-scarum and she had been caught shoplifting, but some years previously she had been seriously injured in a road accident; her younger sister of just under five was worrying her mother because she was so clinging, but the ten other siblings in this family had given no cause for concern. In another family one of the brothers had been fined for throwing stones. Apart from the above two instances there was no known delinquency among the siblings within these five families. They could not be studied in detail, so that other minor behaviour disturbance may have been overlooked, but the general picture was one of uneventful good adjustment, and regular employment in those who had left school.

The Five Children

Janet, at the age of thirteen, was one of a notoriously difficult trio who were a daily trial to their teachers. She had two older sisters, one of whom was a club leader, and six younger siblings, all of whom were stable. A few days before she was born her mother had had to go out in a storm to fetch one of the older children, as a result of which she caught pleurisy and had to be taken to hospital. The mother reported that Janet, unlike all her other children, had never wanted to leave her side when she was a young child. In her later childhood she was quiet and shy, and in recent years had become lazy and listless. At school she showed much hostility towards her teachers, which was reinforced by an anxiety to keep in with her two companions who vied with one another in nuisance value. As a result of the patient diplomacy of the School Welfare Officer all three eventually passed through their difficult phase. Of Janet it was reported that 'She has grown very tall and has settled down well', which suggests that the active phase of her disturbance coincided with the onset of puberty. If it was connected with temporary endocrine imbalance we are still left with the query why this produced instability in this girl and not in most others of her age. Once again we are thrown back upon an individual factor: here, the evidence of Janet's earlier childhood suggests that she had suffered some impairment of temperament which made her susceptible to the endocrine changes of puberty.

Two examples of inconsequence

Hugh was described by his mother at seven years as 'quite a humorous wee boy'. His teachers found him likeable, but a disturber of the peace for whom there seemed no answer. Punishment was no deterrent: he quickly recovered from it, without bearing a grudge. Hugh lacked concentration, did not even try to be neat and tidy, and got very dirty each day in school. Not long back he had fallen into a canal and was pulled out unconscious; but he showed no concern, and soon after regaining consciousness wanted to go out and play again. Nothing made an impression on him; in psychological terms he was impervious to conditioning. His behaviour consisted in a series of responses to immediate situations without regard to the consequences. Like a young puppy he constantly needed petty correction but never remembered for long. What made him such an active nuisance was that he was always on the alert for mischief. He would start off other children in rough play, fool about during team games, misbehave when the teacher was out of the room, accept challenges to perform risky pranks. He was not defective in his needs for personal effectiveness, as is the unforthcoming child, but he satisfied them in a completely moment-to-moment, feckless manner. More children of his type will be met with in the study; we came to call them inconsequential children. Hugh's mother admitted his tiresome ways, describing him as different from her other children. She also mentioned his nervousness and tempers.

He was the ninth of fifteen children, of whom thirteen were still alive. They included the fourteen-year-old girl who had been caught shoplifting, and it is of interest that she was just as inconsequential and unpredictable as he. The mother complained that during her pregnancies she suffered from an asthma-like choking sensation which affected her vocal cords, and it is understandable that she did not welcome her pregnancies beyond the fifth or sixth. Nevertheless, all the children were accepted well when they arrived, and she was an affectionate mother to them. During the eighth month of the pregnancy leading to Hugh's birth she reported that while having two teeth out by gas she did not fully lose consciousness, but that thereafter the dentist had trouble in bringing her round. It is possible that with her tendency to choke she and the foetus suffered some hypoxia. It is unlikely that she emphasized this incident retrospectively in view of the child's defect, because she did not regard him as suffering from anything serious. Moreover, when asked at the beginning of the interview what she thought was the cause of his being 'different' she could give no answer. The dental episode was elicited by a question during a structured interview.

The only defect noted in this boy other than that of temperament was his mumbling, incoherent speech. But late-pregnancy stress could not cause physical malformation, nor proneness to disease unless by damage to reflexes such as those that keep the bronchial tubes clear.

Leslie, at the age of fourteen, showed a very similar pattern of temperamental defect. At school he lacked concentration, disturbed the rest of the class, was a 'show-off', misbehaved when the teacher was out of the room, and constantly needed correction. The School Welfare Officer said of him that 'He never did anything serious but got in the black books of every teacher'. His nervous condition made it impracticable to use corporal punishment on him; he was a bad nailbiter and a finger-sucker; and, like Hugh, had thick, mumbling speech (having had a more serious speech defect when younger). At home he had a similar over-reactivity, being described by his mother as sometimes very irritable, sensitive, and easily upset. The telltale datum, however, was that following a fracture of his skull at seven years he had become mildly epileptic. In this case the unconditionability or inconsequence could be related to evidence of brain damage.

An affectionless character

Alec is of interest as affording an example of the 'affectionless character' or 'moral defective'. It was not that he did not know the difference between right and wrong. He knew that adults took strong exception to stealing, but this only made him more calculating. He stole a money-box from a nursery school, and maintained his denial of the theft with cool lies until he had been identified by several women. A scout himself, he led a gang in breaking into a scout hut. In the course of the subsequent investigation his gambit was, 'I can't understand why you're questioning me'. From a grocer for whom he worked he stole whisky and exchanged it for cakes with some lads who worked in a bakery. He was not prosecuted because he was illegally employed on licensed premises. He also took £1 from the grocer's till, no doubt reckoning that the loss of the note would be regarded as someone's error. He stole repeatedly both in and out of school, and from his own home, but always escaped being charged: he was 'such a nice wee boy'.

He was not a constant nuisance in school as were the last two boys. On the contrary he was 'a charming rogue', glib and plausible, and knowing how to manipulate personal relationships. He even knew how to behave better after being corrected. But the teachers felt that there was always trouble brewing with him – some new act of thieving or spitefulness to weaker children. He would brag and play the hero – using other boys as a foil for his effectiveness needs – but he was indifferent to friendship.

The personality defect from which he suffered was, in sum, a lack of feeling for human attachments and consequently a lack of the anxiety about maintaining good relationships that is the foundation of good conduct. He could not be conditioned to rectitude because there was nothing to appeal to in him: approval was no reward and disapproval no punishment.

How did the devil get into his soul? His mother said that the trouble started when he was six years old, with the birth of a brother. But this event merely provided him with an opportunity for the spitefulness which he exercised upon his younger siblings. A type of maladjustment that consisted in a defect of 'moral sense' would not attract much attention before this age, or at any rate the misdemeanours would not have been regarded very seriously except when they took the form of being spiteful to the baby. This kind of behaviour towards younger children is a constant feature of the affectionless, K-type child,* even though there is little active hostility. Just as a toddler[66] or an ape[34] will enjoy the feeling of effectiveness that comes of reducing an object to small pieces – until the destructiveness is checked by disapproval – so children often seek effectiveness by a 'one-up-manship' at the expense of others. Such behaviour is also held in check by retaliation and the threat of unpopularity, provided the child is sensitive to peer relationships. Spitefulness may just be the exercise of effectiveness or dominance without any such inhibition.

The fact that the mother made the excuse for this boy that he took the arrival of a brother badly is a measure of her stability and tolerance. She admitted that he was 'different' from her other six children, and she was not blind to his bad ways, but there was no hint of her rejecting him. The father had become disgusted with him. He told the headmaster 'You can use the cat o'nine tails if you like'. But such antagonism is understandable so long as the symptoms that the child showed were construed as wilfulness rather than as a distressing form of temperamental handicap. In any case the father's attitude was the result of the behaviour and not the cause of it.

Alec was a restless sleeper and a frequent bedwetter. It was not possible to obtain a systematic account of his early development, but the mother had been very ill following his birth, and there consequently might have been some complication that had affected the child. There was certainly no deprivation of maternal love or care such as might conceivably have produced an incapacity for affection. Jealousy of a younger sibling can never be accepted as an explanation of maladjustment in view of the number of children who do not become jealous, or, if they do, quickly adapt themselves under the

* For the types of maladjustment, see Chapter Nine and Appendix II.

threat of maternal disapproval. It must be viewed as a presenting symptom.

None of the six siblings had given cause for serious concern. The four brothers were described as 'cocky' and one was involved in a fight after he left school; their pattern of life was one of a healthy normal assertiveness. For an explanation of the 'affectionless' character of one member of the family we are left only with the possibility of some congenital neural damage, with which the enuresis and restless sleep would be consistent. This would mean some impairment of the structures that make a person alert to human attachments and induce anxiety when they are endangered.

A 'lazy' boy

Malcolm shared many of the characteristics of the previous three boys. He pilfered money and food from his home and seemed unconcerned about adult approval. His teacher described him as being too immature to heed correction. He showed off, would not attend or concentrate, and was impulsive and easily led into trouble. Once when the School Welfare Officer was in the home talking to his mother the boy burst in with some story to tell, and she had to calm him down by explaining that they had a caller. In a boy of thirteen such a failure to take account of a situation must be reckoned as abnormal. His unconditionability was causing a certain amount of minor domestic trouble: his constant prattle and annoying eating habits incensed the elder brothers and they were ashamed to bring visitors into the home. So inconsequential was Malcolm's behaviour that his parents were worried as to what job he would be capable of, and the father was proposing to get a smallholding which he might later take over.

For both the inconsequential boys described above the teachers had marked the item 'Slumps, lolls about' on the Bristol Guides. For Malcolm, in the section for 'Favourite Activity' his teacher had written 'Too lazy to have *any* interest in *any* physical activity'. At team games he was dreamy and uninterested, always sluggish, lethargic, timid, and poor-spirited. He could never find any activity with which to amuse himself, since he had no interests. He had a beggar mentality: having spent the money for his fares to and from school he cadged off passers-by in the street. He exploited his simpleness by assuming the role of the stupid clown; at home he also 'played daft' and put on physical incapacities. With the School Welfare Officer he tried to ingratiate himself by telling self-pitying yarns, pleading the rightness of his behaviour, and drawing attention to the faults of his classmates. His only delinquencies were that he obtained some cigarettes by fraud and was once charged with throwing stones.

In terms of the theory of behaviour outlined in a later chapter this boy seemed to suffer from a double personality defect. He was content to be a thoroughly ineffective person. If this had been the only thing wrong with him he would have been an unassertive, unforthcoming child. In addition, he seemed to have something of the impairment of the previous case: not only was there little instinctive need for effectiveness or self-respect; he had little sense of personal attachment that might form the basis for social conditioning. He was motivated neither by his own pride nor by the desire for approval. Thus he became a 'lazy' boy.

It would once again be too far-fetched to seek the causes of these personality defects in his upbringing. His three brothers were stable, their only delinquency being that one of them had been charged, like him, with throwing stones. The father was commendably tolerant, and the mother was found by the Welfare Officer to be very understanding.

She related that all her children had been born rapidly and without assistance. The birth of this child was proceeding well and, indeed, too rapidly to allow the trainee nurse time to come and attend it – whereupon the Sister attempted to delay the delivery by pushing against the head until the trainee could arrive. In the hospital the mother suspected that something was wrong because the baby never cried. He also seemed to have some neural insensitivity, for he would lie with a corner of the pillow pressing into his eye. He remained an unduly placid baby. At the age of thirteen he suffered from chronic mild upper respiratory disease and poor muscular coordination, and held his body in an unnatural posture as if slightly spastic.

Of these five children, despite their instability and nuisance value, only one was a persistent delinquent, and he of a special type suggesting unconcern for good human relationships rather than anxiety. Considering how tiresome and emotionally unrewarding these children must have been to their parents, the latter exercised unusual tolerance, and the family situations may also be accounted unusually free of stress. One suspects that these temperamentally susceptible children were preserved from more serious behavioural breakdown because they were thus protected.

Possible Explanations of Behaviour Disturbance

Congenital impairment

Apart from being members of stable families and having siblings of more than average stability, the salient feature among the five was somatic and/or neural impairment. Two were enuretic, one was epileptic, three had speech defects, and two had unnatural bodily posture. It is hard to escape the impression that their disturbed behaviour sprang from an impairment of the neural structures, which could also have been congenital. In three of the five cases there had been a report by the mother of some complication during the pregnancy or birth; in another a birth complication was possible. The fifth case was that of the epileptic boy with a speech defect and slight spastic condition in whom brain injury must be assumed. These factors, such as they could be ascertained, are summarized in *Table 1.*

Stresses in the school situation

As an alternative to the stresses of the family situation must be considered those that arise within the school itself. From the point of view of the prevention and reduction of behaviour disturbance this is an important consideration, and it is discussed in a later chapter. It is quite feasible, and indeed only to be anticipated, that the degree of stress within the school situation will influence the total incidence of delinquency and other evidence of disturbance. Nevertheless, it could not account for the maladjustment of these five children since the assessment of their maladjustment was made by teachers in relation to the general behaviour of a whole class of children. If a few reacted by disturbed behaviour there must have been reasons for such a differential reaction. The practical criterion for maladjustment is an aberrant reaction to situations in which the majority behave in a stable manner.

Backwardness

The same applies to responses to particular stressful experiences, either within the school or elsewhere. It may for instance be asked to what extent the maladjustment of these five children was due to backwardness and its attendant frustrations and sense of failure. Since they were in non-academic types of school there were many other pupils whose attainment was poor and no undue emphasis was placed upon competitive standards. A somewhat backward child

Table 1 Five disturbed children in stable, non-stressful families

Name	*Age*	*BSAG score**	*Delinquency*	*No. of siblings*	*Behaviour of siblings*	*Somatic and neural impairment*	*Congenital factors*
Janet	13	22	None	8	All stable	Enuresis	Mother contracted pleurisy shortly before confinement
Hugh	7	23	None	12	All stable except for inconsequential sister caught shoplifting and clinging pre-school sister	Slight speech defect	Pregnancy unwanted; asthma-like choking; complication in administration of gas in dental operation
Leslie	14	37	None	2	Both stable	Epilepsy; unnatural posture; speech defect (skull fracture at 7 years); bad nailbiter	
Alec	13	18	Persistent	6	All stable	Enuresis, restless sleep	Mother very ill as a result of his birth
Malcolm	13	35	Minor	3	All stable	Neural insensitivity and failure to cry as a baby; upper respiratory infections; poor muscular coordination; unnatural posture; speech defect; fat	Delivery artificially delayed to enable trainee nurse to attend

* The number of indications of maladjustment recorded on the Bristol Social Adjustment Guides

would not therefore feel an undue sense of failure or be subjected to pressure.

The teachers were asked to assess the attainments of the children in reading and arithmetic on a four-point scale consisting of 'good', 'average', 'poor for age', 'cannot read' or 'completely incompetent' (arithmetic). The fourth category was marked for only one of the five (Leslie), in respect of his performance in arithmetic, and he was also 'poor' at reading; this boy had a history of epilepsy and speech defect. Of the ten possible ratings, seven were 'average' and one 'good'. There is consequently no reason for attributing the behaviour disturbance of this group of five children to particular frustrations arising from their school work.

'Cultural' maladjustment

A further alternative explanation of maladjustment, which has some currency at present, is that it is not due to emotional disturbance or personality defect, but is merely the normal mode of behaviour of children coming from certain subcultures. To this the same general answer may be given: the non-academic secondary schools in question drew their children from culturally homogeneous areas, so that the types of behaviour rated as disturbed were differential reactions. This is not to say that certain children who have been brought up to a way of life that places little emphasis upon schooling will not meet certain difficulties in adaptation, especially when they are eager to leave school and start earning. But the fact is that the great majority of such children adapt themselves well to what has to be. It is also a cardinal principle of the traditional non-aspiring, hedonistic pattern of culture that good face-to-face relationships should be maintained with those people with whom the individual is in daily contact. In his study of schoolchildren from an underprivileged quarter of Liverpool, Mays[39] comments upon the good relationships between teachers and children. From discussion with the School Welfare Officers the writer ascertained that the same applied to these Glasgow schools. In no case, despite pointed inquiry, could any hint be elicited of a teacher's provoking a child to any exceptional behavioural reaction or of any other particular stressful situation. In fact, owing to the presence of the School Welfare Officer within each school, these children must have found some mitigation of the normal degree of stress and a safety valve for their difficulties. The fact, therefore, that some of them differed from the rest of their class in having bad relationships with their teachers, or in causing them trouble, points to some individual cause outside the school and untypical of their cultural background. There is, however, no intention of writing down the general influence of the culture; it is a powerful one, but acts in other and more important ways than by a direct imprinting of norms of conduct upon the child.[73]

CHAPTER TWO

Children with a Degree of Stressful Family Experience

In this chapter will be discussed the group of eleven children who found themselves in somewhat stressful family situations, together with two who had lost their mothers during their earlier childhood. In none of these cases, however, did the contemporary situation or the situation that had obtained for the past nine or ten years reach the critical level of stress characteristic of the standard maladjustment-conducive patterns. This assessment is supported by the evidence that there were only four delinquent or unstable children out of a total of fifty-one known full siblings in the thirteen families.

Characteristics of the Family Situations

Low stress-tolerance and over-reactivity

Geoffrey was described by his mother as always having been 'different' from her other seven well-behaved children. He was sensitive, easily upset, subject to terrible tempers, awkward, generally tiresome, and allowed himself to be dared into risky pranks. From just before eight years he had a history of repeated truancy and shoplifting, to which at thirteen years he added the theft of a cycle and housebreaking.

In the section of the Bristol Guide for 'Favourite Activity' his teacher wrote, 'Making himself a nuisance'. His maladjustment was predominantly of the hostile type, but with an admixture of attention-seeking, showing off, moodiness, and distractability.

With a maladjustment score of 35 and an 82 per cent prognosis of delinquency on the Prediction Instrument, it was evident that the boy's general temperamental susceptibility had been aggravated by a stressful situation. Until he was eight, the parents with their four children lived in a single room and indeed slept in one bed. Geoffrey spent much time with a grandmother who lived near by, whose home, one gathered, served as a refuge for him from the stresses of overcrowded living. When the family moved to the luxury of two rooms in another district he was deprived of such relief, and the overcrowding must have been little less harassing since, in the meantime, three more children had been born, and twins were shortly to arrive.

The mother kept her household and her family well organized, and worked during the weekends as a waitress. She thrashed Geoffrey if he stayed out late, but tended to spoil the younger children. In her attempts to discipline him she also used threats to have him put away. The School Welfare Officer was rightly convinced that these were not seriously uttered; to an emotionally robust child they would no doubt have been taken lightheartedly but to the over-sensitized, stress-vulnerable boy they were evidently construed as rejection. He also showed indubitable symptoms of anxiety, continually giving his mother presents and making things for her, and – apparently from his odd earnings – giving her more money than she wanted to take from him. Evidently he feared the possibility of being 'put away', and this would account for his persistent truancy (once staying out all night), his delinquencies, and his hostility to adults.

The mother was very angry at the pregnancy because it came too soon after the last, quite apart from the overcrowded conditions. As a baby Geoffrey slept so continuously that, in her words, 'We didn't know the colour of his eyes for eleven months'. As a toddler he became a wanderer, which indicates impairment of the instinctive attachment mechanisms. During all his childhood he was a restless sleeper and enuretic.

This case, in summary, conformed to the pattern of the five described in the previous chapter, with the history of early impairment and disorganized behaviour of the inconsequential and over-reacting type; but, given a certain amount of family insecurity and stress, the temperamental susceptibility flared up into open delinquency and other waywardness.

Four other cases show so similar a pattern of low stress-tolerance, inconsequence, or over-reaction that they can be dealt with together. In all four, also, the mother had to a degree lost patience with the child and had threatened 'putting away'. Three of them had stable siblings. Of *Duncan* the mother said, 'With just this boy things seem to have gone wrong'. *Mary*'s behaviour at home caused tremendous flare-ups and her mother had got to the stage where she wanted to get rid of her. Mary herself came to the School Welfare Officer saying she wanted to leave home; if she was not taken away she would steal something from a shop and get put away. *Roger*'s mother had not fully recovered from the death of her husband two years earlier, and was economically harassed; she likewise threatened to have the boy removed from home if he gave further trouble. He was subject to tantrums, and in addition annoyed his mother by wanting to spend holidays with a former woman neighbour whom she accused of having made a fuss of him when he was young. His hankering after her did not seem to justify the description of divided maternal attachment that was appropriate for some children in the next group. But it seemed to be enough to estrange his relations with his mother somewhat in her overwrought state. *Albert*'s parents were chronic quarrellers but the Welfare Officer felt that, with them, this was a mode of living; they were fond of each other, and did not allow the family stresses to get to the point of disintegration. Nevertheless, the effect of such an atmosphere with five people living in one room was that the elder sister had become unstable and erratic, and the elder brother delinquent. Albert was quite unable to bear the chronic stress and strain of the bickering family. He ran away four or five times, and gave way to irresponsible outbursts.

All four children had a history of illness or neural impairment. Duncan had had tuberculosis at eleven years. Mary suffered from 'black-outs'; examination at one hospital suggested epilepsy but at another no definite diagnosis could be made. Roger weighed $10\frac{1}{2}$ lbs at birth – which is in the high-risk class[32] – and the labour was long and difficult. On coming to live in the city at eleven years he developed an intolerance of noises. At thirteen he was very scared of dental treatment and afraid to go far from home, to enter the local shop, or to go on buses alone. He was gawky and 'chesty', thin, and extremely pale. Albert had had a convulsive fit as a baby which was almost fatal and other minor attacks during his first two years. As a toddler he was a wanderer, and tiresome and destructive. His speech was described as of the 'scrambled eggs' variety; he was gawky, and his nervous mannerisms made his mother think he had St Vitus's Dance. He had a great aversion to being touched upon the face or neck. Roger and he showed rather a similar neural impairment, which might be characterized as low stress-tolerance and inability to inhibit diversions and discomfort.

Three 'vulnerable' children

Rose's hostility to the adult world was so active (of a total maladjustment score of 36, 11 items were for hostility) that she got the whole of the staff against her. The Welfare Officer reported, 'I cannot explain how bad things were at school; everyone heaved a sigh of relief when she left.' For hostility of this degree one expects to find some urgent reason in the contemporary home situation. The parents' marriage had been a short and unhappy one, the father deserting when Rose was three. A very difficult great-aunt who lived with the family became antagonistic to her. Evidently the great-aunt played the part of the rejecting father of pattern F, who brings pressure to have the child put away. Nevertheless there seemed no real danger of the mother succumbing to any such pressure. She admitted that her daughter had got on her nerves with her tiresome ways and she vacillated between defence and rejection. Rose was very defiant to her mother and moody and deceitful at home. There were in effect indications that things sometimes got to the pass where the mother would support the great-aunt's rejection.

There was one elder brother, who was stable, with a good employment record. Before one simply blames the great-aunt as an insecurity-producing factor one must ask why she became antagonistic to the girl. It could have been that some initial behaviour disturbance underlay the intolerance. The only indications of somatic or neural impairment in the girl were that she was a restless sleeper, was jumpy, and had protruding eyes that suggested exophthalmic goitre.

Herbert, a youngest child with four stable elder brothers, all of whom had married and were living away from the family home, was another case that suggested neural impairment. The only concomitant defect was his thick, mumbling speech; but he showed the typical combination of low stress-tolerance and inconsequence. He was an indiscriminate attention-seeker, sidling up to and hanging round his teacher, tiring with constant chatter and sulking if he did not get attention. He disturbed other children's games, hurt and frightened them by petty molestation, and flew into tempers. He had the usual inconsequential showing off and hero-playing. But his nervous resources were poor: he scored eight indications for depression, including wandering off alone and solitary truancy. His mother said that, apart from a delinquent friend he had had at one time, he never mixed much with other children, liked staying indoors, and had to be made to go out. However, this abnormality saved him from delinquency despite a high prediction score.

His own father had been killed at work when he was quite young. Between three and five years he attended a nursery school, where he was described as neglected and the mother as uncooperative. One might surmise that, as so often occurs, she partially went to pieces after the death of her husband. Her second marriage was an unhappy one; she spoke disparagingly of her present husband, declaring that she stayed with him only for the boy's sake. With the antagonism that would thus have been generated between the boy and his stepfather, such a situation would have been stressful. The mother's loyalty to him prevented it from falling into one of the standard maladjustment-inducing patterns. But the combination of temperamental vulnerability and chronic stress made a maladjusted boy.

Stewart's mother made a wartime marriage while in her teens, but for five years she had no children, and since her husband was found to be consorting with other women there was a separation. Some time after he was called up he announced to her that he had had a son by another woman and asked her to take him. She was sorry for the baby, and did so. During the war the husband was twice convicted of bigamy, but she nevertheless eventually took him back and had two sons by him, of whom Stewart was the younger. During the pregnancy the husband was found to be having relations with yet another woman, and when the child was two years old he deserted for good.

The informally adopted boy proved a great standby to her and she became deeply devoted to him. As for her own two boys, they were the sons of the husband whom she regretted re-accepting, and she regretted having them also. The elder of the two had in fact never given much trouble except for a phase of refusal to attend school at the primary stage, and they were both well-behaved and considerate at home. She had suffered from nervous trouble from shortly after the temporary return of her husband, and was prematurely aged. It was unfortunate that she lived in a council estate notorious for the social deviance of the tenants, and those upstairs drove her to desperation by their noisy bottle parties. She had developed paranoiac tendencies, isolating herself from neighbours, wanting to keep her curtains closed during the day and going out as little as possible. During her unbalanced chattering she would predict being in the cemetery in a few months, saying this in front of her sons. The elder said he did not worry about it, she was always talking like that and did not mean any of it.

As for Stewart, he showed some anxiety symptoms over his mother. His teacher gave a very bad report on his behaviour and he could not be got to concentrate on anything. He was very nervous, never smiled, and talked ceaselessly. Although getting a high delinquency-prediction score he committed only one minor offence, that of breaking windows with other boys when he was ten years old, which would hardly have been deviant behaviour in his neighbourhood. His mother said that he had always been nervous and fidgety, and while at the primary school he had been referred to the child guidance clinic. The wonder is that he and his brother did not show more maladjustment than they did. Possibly the 'brother', who was some years older than they, provided a stable element in their lives and helped them to ignore the mother's irresponsible talk. No doubt also she was not completely an unreliable mother in fact. Certainly she had been soft-hearted enough to her husband and to the baby he brought home for her to rear.

A case of maternal deprivation?

Carol was the second of the troublesome trio mentioned in the previous chapter. Her parents had deserted their family within a short time of each other, when Carol was four years old. With her four elder siblings and two younger cousins (whose parents also deserted) she was taken in by the grandparents who lived in the flat above. When the mother was getting herself ready for the final parting she dressed Carol, her youngest, to take with her, but the grandmother intervened and the mother acquiesced without putting up much resistance. Since the little girl had been constantly in her mother's company until the parting this experience must have been a traumatic one at the time, for which she later may unconsciously have blamed the grandmother.

The point of interest in this case is why this girl alone of the seven abandoned children showed any instability. The grandmother was a very determined and dominant woman, rather rough in her dealings with people and inclined to be 'anti-school' – the kind of person in short who would have been likely to utter insensitive threats of 'putting away'. The fact remains, however, that she acted as a very effective surrogate mother for her two families of grandchildren. One must suppose that if Carol's childhood experience had a lasting adverse effect it was either because the trauma occurred at a critical age or because she was unduly susceptible to stress. She was enuretic and a restless sleeper, extremely labile of mood and prone to tempers, but usually quiet, 'shut in', and very shy with strangers.

It may have been, on the other hand, that the loss of her mother some nine years back had little connection with her behaviour disturbance. This, which consisted of active hostility and a settled rejection of her teachers (types HA and K) together with an anxiety to keep in with her troublesome friends (XC), was very similar to that of her friend Janet, who had suffered no early maternal deprivation.

All one can say is that here were two thirteen-year-old girls, both enuretic, who were quiet and shy at home but troublesome in school, without there being any evidently stressful contemporary home situation. The third of the trio – to be described later – certainly had a bad family background, and it may have been that she introduced the pattern of hostility and rejection that the others copied. This does not of course explain why they, of all the girls in the class, should have done so.

Avoidance delinquency

Andrew had been a wanderer from infancy, his mother reporting that it was difficult to keep him in the house. All his five siblings were normal, the two elder sisters being described as outstandingly superior girls. At home he was moody, easily upset, did not have a civil word for any of his family, set out to annoy, never smiled, was deceitful, and had terrible tempers during which he would throw things. He truanted and stayed away from home for hours, spending his time doing odd jobs for other people, while refusing to run errands for his mother. The family had immigrated from Malta when he was four; but he said that he hated the Maltese and liked the Scots. This unusual antipathy to members of his own race offered a clue, and it was suspected that the mother, in her exasperation, had been threatening to send him back to Malta if he did not mend his ways. When, following the case conference, the mother was revisited, she admitted that she had frequently done so. The boy confirmed this, saying that at first he thought she was joking, but latterly had been worried about it. Once this unwitting cause of the hostility was removed he became 'a different boy'.

Nonetheless, such neat psychological solutions of behaviour disturbance must be accepted with reserve, and only when supported by strong evidence. One has to ask why this particular boy took so seriously threats of a type that many an exasperated mother may utter from time to time. Moreover, his response to the anxiety that it caused him was the extreme one of unconscious avoidance, with all that that entails in the form of irrational behaviour. To keep the threat to his insecurity from his mind he needed to resort to compulsive acts and substitutive emotional tensions. His delinquencies answered to the well-established pattern of excitement-seeking as a means of escaping from a haunting anxiety.[56] He snatched food from shops, stole lead from church roofs, and once broke into a church. The stolen goods, having served their purpose, were given away to friends. Such an inability to tolerate anxiety suggests some temperamental frailty.

Stanley's delinquency was also motivated by avoidance-excitement. He gave little trouble in school and his teachers could report few indications of behaviour disturbance in him for the simple reason that he was seldom there. In his efforts to keep his anxieties from intruding into his conscious mind the pathological avoider seeks an endless succession of new sensations. Consciousness is reduced to perception, with the occasional addition of realistic fantasy. The sameness of a schoolroom or a factory workshop becomes intolerable, the victim complaining that he cannot stand being shut in and must be in the open air. With a truanting gang Stanley made repeated excursions to Edinburgh, some forty-five miles from his home, and other places outside Glasgow, committing minor delinquencies on the way. He could never stay a moment in his own home, even when he managed to avoid school with the excuse of a sore eye or similar incapacity. If, when running past a shop, he presumably sensed some reminder of his anxiety, he would dive in and grab something.

His truancy and delinquency began when a younger brother was killed by a van outside their house. The mother, who saw the dead child soon after the accident, was badly affected and suffered what was virtually a nervous breakdown. She became intolerant of Stanley and several times demanded of the School Welfare Officer that she get him removed. In court, however, both she and the boy were greatly distressed when the removal became a reality. Her rejection was an instance of the irritable-depressive non-tolerance, typical of breakdown under stress. In his approved school, away from reminders of his insecurity, the boy seemed happy, with no yearning for travel. But he had nightmares of seeing a 'green lady' (Health Visitor) walking across the room. No doubt the Health Visitor had frequent occasion to call following the accident in view of the mother's state and her numerous young children.

There can be no doubt that the triggering-off cause of Stanley's waywardness was the death of his brother two and a half years back and the consequent nervous shock to his mother. But once again we have to beware of neat, self-contained explanations. It must be asked why the behaviour of his ten younger siblings remained unaffected by their mother's condition, and why she turned against him. Unfortunately, within the limits of the School Welfare Officers' work it was not possible to follow up these cases as aetiological studies in order to try to get the answers to questions such as these. We can only surmise that, like the others discussed above, he was a stress-vulnerable child.

Neil's mother died of cancer when he was six. After her death the father went out drinking every night, leaving the children unattended. Three years later he remarried, but the boy refused to accept his stepmother, although she was a warm-hearted woman who was patient and tried her best with him. This was the most striking instance in this series where unconscious avoidance of a traumatic experience resulted in behavioural aberration. Even before he was of an age to be charged in court Neil took to housebreaking, and received his first conviction for this offence at the age of ten. The beltings that he received from his father only had the effect of making him stay away from home. When he was twelve, while playing truant, the police caught him throwing bottles at passing cars. He did not come home that evening, and his stepmother, going out to search for him, found him after midnight, soaking wet, huddled in a midden. For some unknown reason he wanted to keep pigeons, but was charged with wilful cruelty to a pigeon in the street. After several appearances in court he was committed to twenty-eight days' detention and finally to an approved school. He was in fact typical of the many avoidance-excitement cases that find their way, undiagnosed, into approved schools.*

How near to psychosis Neil had been driven by the compulsion to blot out the traumatic memory of his mother's death is illustrated by an incident when he was somewhat younger. While his stepmother

* Many cases are described in detail in the writer's report to the Carnegie United Kingdom Trust, *Delinquency and Human Nature*.[55] There was evidence of avoidance-excitement being the direct motivation of their delinquency in 55 of the 102 cases studied.

was putting him to bed he asked to go to the toilet; half an hour later he was brought back by the police, having been found wandering in a public park. The unconscious avoidance remained active six years after the death of his mother; asked if he ever thought of her, his face crumpled up just as if he might cry but without apparent emotion, and he said, 'There is too much to do, there's no time to think.' It would be difficult to obtain a clearer introspection of the refusal to face a traumatic memory. The starting-point of the avoider's behavioural aberrations is that he cannot bear to be left with any unoccupied thinking time.

As often happens in these cases the pattern of hectic, irresponsible hyperactivity was superimposed upon an otherwise well-adjusted personality. Neil was described by the stepmother as a very good boy in the house, and her two baby girls worshipped him. Similarly, at school he presented no disciplinary problem, and indeed his conduct was reported to be excellent. This was confirmed by his low score of six on the Bristol Guides; the only adverse items were his truancy, damage to public property, and a certain aloofness from teachers, who noted that he said very little and seldom smiled. The report on his period in the remand home ran as follows: 'During his stay here he kept himself clean and tidy. His relationships with the staff were good and he created a very favourable impression. He was amenable to discipline and generally helpful and eager to please. Full of life, he is continually on the go and always on the look-out for adventure (*sic*). In class he was the same brisk, bright little boy causing no trouble whatever. He worked well, within his capacities, and could be relied on to do his work without constant driving.' In just over a year after his release from detention he was in an approved school for theft.

His case prompts an important reflection concerning the relationship between delinquency and maladjustment: it can by no means be assumed that all the delinquent children making low scores on the Bristol Guides are free from behaviour disturbance. Such scores are the result of observation of the child within a particular environment.* Attitudes of hostility or rejection are often transferred from one human situation to another, and attention-seeking, inhibited, and inconsequential children usually reveal themselves in all situations. With avoidance-excitement, however, the child – as in the case of Neil – may be quite normal in an environment that keeps him occupied and contains no reminders of the dreaded memory. In other

* A series of careful case studies should be made of apparently stable delinquent children.

cases the child may take refuge in realistic fantasy and show no behaviour disturbance in school except chronic day-dreaming; in yet others, the demand for substitutive sensation may be so impelling that the child cannot tolerate the sameness of any enclosed surroundings and has to roam, like Cain fleeing the memory of his brother's murder. Neil's truancy and nocturnal wandering were probably thus motivated.

His case poses a final query. Why should it be that he reacted by such extreme avoidance to the loss of his mother, whereas so many other similarly bereaved children remain unaffected once the grief has been worked through? Why did his younger brother – who was about four when the mother died – accept the warm-hearted stepmother and he not? Any such differences of reaction might be explained by postulating a critical age at which the deprivation becomes traumatic. But there have been many changes of opinion as to which is the critical age. The Kleinians originally put it in the first six months of life. In Hilda Lewis's study of children taken into care,[35] the group who showed most subsequent maladjustment were those separated from their parents after the age of five years. If we say that, with the present family in mind, six may be a more vulnerable age than four, we are reminded of the troublesome Carol, who was four years old when her mother deserted. Both she and Neil had been very attached to their mothers, and the closeness of the relationship is no doubt a factor. But the intensity of the need for attachment is an individual variable, and the suggestion that common sense advises – until some alternative relationship is established – is that the degree of trauma depends upon the temperament of the individual child. There was little to suggest that Neil was in any way temperamentally impaired, but there may have been some delay in maturation: at nearly thirteen he was described by the School Welfare Officer as 'very small, with a very baby little face'.

A 'cultural' delinquent

Bernard was interesting as a 'cultural' case. Among their other irregular sources of income the family were professional garbage rummagers, doing the rounds of domestic dustbins. Three elder brothers had been delinquent, an elder sister had engaged in a razor fight, and another – apparently the white sheep of the family – was put out of the house because her boy-friend was disapproved of. To those who like to posit a criminal subculture, in which stable calculating 'businessmen' (good husbands in their time off) follow the trade of crime and bring up their sons to it, this family must have seemed a showcase specimen. But the father was by no means a good family man; he was violent to his children, and had been seen kicking one of his daughters. Nor did Bernard by any means answer to the theoretical type. Far from being the well-adjusted lad who carried the family pattern of sturdy subcultural deviance into school with him, he was timid and poor-spirited, never fighting among other boys, selfish, and a bad loser. His behaviour, with his heedlessness of correction, quick resort to tears, being easily led into mischief, destructiveness, forgetfulness, and lack of consistent incentives, was typical of the pattern of inconsequence. There were also several signs of physical and neural impairment in him – lifelessness, thick inaudible speech, aimless hand movements, asthma, a small puny build.

Nonetheless, this was a 'cultural' case, albeit in a different sense. Such families could not have been good ones by the yardstick of any culture. In similar criminal families studied by the writer,[55] where all the sons as well as the father had had many convictions (cases of Faulkner, Mathews, and Rich), it was clear that at any rate the mothers deplored the manner of life into which their families had fallen. The boys showed intense mother-anxiety, and in one case a pathological flight into a fantasy of an idyllic home. When it was suggested to one of these mothers that her son should be licensed from his approved school to live with his married sister and her husband, she despondently pointed out that they were a cut above them, they were wage-earners. A culture implies a manner of life evolved by a social group because of its survival value; its transmission has conferred a greater safety and skill of living that take the group above the appalling biological wastage of animal existence. In no sense can these criminal families be said to possess a successful culture. Their pattern of life is rather one of cultural disintegration or deprivation, as Wilson[79] points out in reference to the group of 'performance-inadequate' families that she studied.

Even the physical and neural impairments that abound in members of these 'problem' families would seem to be a direct result of the stresses that cultural deprivation entails. With the life that this particular mother had led it is very unlikely that she ever enjoyed a happy, settled pregnancy; it is not surprising that she was bedraggled-looking and in poor health. Under such conditions there would have been a considerable risk of congenital damage to the children. One may ask whether this may not be the common factor underlying the feeblemindedness, physical defects, mental illness, and general weakness of character found in the Kallikak-type problem family, which is popularly ascribed to 'bad stock'.

Seven of the thirteen disturbed children discussed in this chapter reacted adversely against threats to being put out of the home, and similar threats may have been made to the others. In all these cases there was a family situation involving a degree of stress, and either it did not bear as hard on the siblings or else they remained unaffected by it. There was reason to believe, from the early indications of behaviour disturbance, that some of these children had by their own instability created stressful situations against themselves. All appeared unusually stress-vulnerable: seven were inconsequential over-reactors, three were impelled by unconscious avoidance of traumatic experience, and one sought physical removal from her stressful home situation.

Prechtl[46] has pointed out, as a difficulty in assessing the effect of maternal deprivation, that the mother's rejection may itself be a reaction to unrewarding behaviour in the infant. A constant screamer may induce compulsive dislike; a failure of attachment behaviour in the form of refusal of endearments, or a hyperactivity that prevents the child from remaining long on the mother's knee, may be resented. Just as the young child gives its affection where it senses the readiest acceptance,[51] so the mother may be expected to lavish her warmest affections upon the child who gives most affection in return. Only the most careful and objective case history-taking can disentangle original cause and effect in such cases.

As in the previous group of cases there is a striking incidence of somatic-neural impairment, affecting eleven of the thirteen children. These included two instances of epilepsy or early convulsions and two of enuresis. The cases are summarized in *Table 2*.

Table 2 Thirteen disturbed children with a degree of stressful family experience

Name	*Age*	*BSAG score*	*Delin-quency*	*No. of siblings*	*Behaviour of siblings*	*Somatic and neural impairment*	*Congenital factors*
Geoffrey	13	35	Persistent	7	Stable	Enuresis, restless sleep; wanderer as toddler	
Duncan	14	31	None	3	Stable	Tuberculosis at 11 years	
Mary	13	25	None	3 (full) 2 (half)	Stable	Epilepsy	
Roger	13	23	Minor	3	Stable	Thin, extremely pale; noise intolerant; poor muscular coordination; upper respiratory infections	Birth weight 10½ lbs; long difficult labour
Albert	13	30	Minor	2	Unstable and delinquent	Early convulsions; wanderer and tiresome as toddler; jumbled speech; athetoid movements; compulsive fears	
Rose	14	36	None	1	Stable	Exophthalmic goitre (?); restless sleep	
Herbert	13	35	None	4	Stable	Imperfect speech	

Stewart	13	?	Minor	1	Unstable	Had always been fidgety and nervous	Husband unfaithful during pregnancy, following two bigamous marriages
Carol	13	25	None	4	All stable	Enuresis, restless sleep	Unstable marriage
Andrew	14	25	Persistent	5	Stable	Wanderer from infancy	
Stanley	14	10*	Persistent	10	Stable		
Neil	13	6	Persistent	3 (full) 2 (half)	All stable	Very small for age; babyish features; headaches, sickness	?
Bernard	14	25	Persistent	5	Four delinquent	Asthma, upper respiratory infections; imperfect speech; athetoid movements; small and very thin	

* Seldom at school owing to truancy and malingering

CHAPTER THREE

Children in Critically Stressful Family Situations

In the remaining fifteen cases in the sample the family situations answered to one or other of the standard maladjustment and delinquency-producing patterns.[56] The common factor in them was their unreliability from the child's point of view. There was a constant danger of their disintegration by the desertion of one or other parent; or the child was under the threat of being put out of the home; or else he had made but was deprived of a primary attachment to a surrogate parent.

These cases will be reviewed with two questions in mind. In the present chapter it will be asked to what extent the maladjustment seems to be the natural consequence – without adducing other variables – of the child's family circumstances; and, as a corollary, whether the type of maladjustment can be matched with the type of familial insecurity. In the following chapter will be discussed to what extent the stressful family situations resulted from wider cultural stresses.

The Family Patterns

Parental quarrelling

The most frequent of these pathological family situations was pattern A – that of parental quarrelling so severe as to threaten the continued existence of the marriage partnership. In each case the marital disharmony centred on some misconduct or inadequacy of one of the marriage partners.

In the case of *Desmond* it was his stepmother's conduct that was the source of the trouble. The father suspected her of 'carrying on' with a young lad, and rushing home one day found the youth in his home. His wife's becoming pregnant increased his suspicions, and he set his son to watch his mother. The boy complained that for dinner he got only a roll and tea, while the boy-friend got the good food. He also said that his parents quarrelled over money, and the family did seem in fact to be in financial difficulties because the gas had been cut off. Both parents had threatened to desert, and after one row the father talked of suicide.

The boy's maladjustment as seen in school was the expected one of extreme hostility (13 indications, mostly at the severe end of the hostility scale). He had been put out of various classes and was convinced that the whole staff, including the headmaster, were down on him. At times, no doubt during family crises, he showed symptoms of compulsive avoidance behaviour, careering around the school wildly. He behaved notably badly towards the women teachers, and in his primary school used to punch girls in the playground. At home, however, he made surprisingly mature attempts to alleviate the situation. He retained a certain amount of faith in his father, whom he helped in his street-trading job. Out of his not inconsiderable earnings he once gave his mother £5, and was extremely generous to a neighbour's children. At school also he was described as a tender-hearted, kindly boy, which tends to confirm that his earlier ill treatment of girls had had a compulsive motivation. He had been convicted, during his mother's illicit affair, of housebreaking with four other boys; for this he was given a deferred sentence, and a fine of £7 was imposed on his father. But the boy paid the fine out of his earnings. As a measure of his contradictory honesty, he collected all his father's accounts when the latter was ill, amounting to £150 at the weekend, and handed over the money entire.

The degree of conflict to which he was subjected evoked the typical urge to remove himself from the stressful situation. He was keen to be sent away to a residential school in order, as he put it, to get away from teachers and people who bossed him about; but he did not want to go until after Christmas, because he hoped that his parents' quarrelling would cease by then. Unfortunately he was refused a month's stay in such a school owing to his tendency to black-outs and dizzy turns. This refusal produced a renewed outbreak of bad behaviour.

Apart from the black-outs, which he had had only in recent years, he was also a bedwetter and restless sleeper, and subject to nervous mannerisms. Such symptoms are not unusual in states of extreme emotional stress, so that one must suppose them to be a psychosomatic reaction thereto. It is, however, idle to try to decide whether they are environmental or congenital, since they must be a combination of both: once the stress-tolerance threshold has been overstepped the form of the breakdown will be determined by the somatic and emotional weaknesses to which the individual is constitutionally subject. For this reason we can never expect to find a complete talliance between the type of stressful situation and the response to it.

The degree of stress to which *Samuel* was subjected can be judged by the reactions of his siblings: one elder brother was in an approved school, another in a mental institution by a court order, and a younger sister lived with a grandmother. There were another four younger siblings of whom nothing adverse had so far been reported. The father spent much of his day in bed, being found thus even in the late afternoon by the Probation Officer. After five years of mostly voluntary idleness he obtained a temporary job, but worked for only two weeks of the possible four and left owing his employer money. He spent on drink what money he could lay his hands on, and had deserted for a period during which he cohabited with another woman. He was finally convicted of assaulting his wife. The latter, though she had resigned herself to his work shyness, had also deserted the home for some three months and was considering a legal separation.

At school the boy scored no fewer than 58 indications of behaviour disturbance. Among these were high hostility (13), as would be anticipated with such a degree of insecurity, and also high K (9 indications), a more set rejection of adults which in the circumstances might be no less expected. His behaviour deteriorated markedly at the time of his father's imprisonment for wife-assault. In trying to convince a teacher of his innocence over some misdemeanour he became quite hysterical as if he had no recollection of it himself. He contracted severe migrainous headaches and complained of stomach pains and feeling sick.

Like the previous boy the possibility of being removed from the home did not worry him, and his delinquency – breaking into premises – was probably motivated by the chance it offered of escape from his stressful situation.

Jean's father was also a non-worker, and spent his National Assistance money on smoking and drink. The mother never had a good word for him and complained that he had recently given her an awful beating up. But she was equally unbalanced, and periodically went into hospital for mental treatment. She had deserted and returned to the home several times. Surprisingly, the girl showed little hostility; she seemed on the contrary quite phlegmatic. Her behaviour was not unduly bad, but her attitude to the staff was one of detachment without the least desire to please. Yet she was remarkably neat and clean in her work, and her attainment was good considering her lack of need for approval. She was spiteful and unkind to her younger brother and sister, and her mother complained that she was 'cold' and that one did not know how to take her. As a young child she was tiresome and destructive. At fourteen she was stocky and very fat, and a restless sleeper. One suspects that she was saved from anxiety by an impairment of her attachment needs. But her need for personal effectiveness was apparently unimpaired: despite her unprepossessing appearance she followed the extravagant *bouffant* hair style of the adolescents of her generation and was described as a typical Teddy girl. Being so emotionally self-contained she had not the resentment against her insecurity that might have impelled her towards social deviance.

We have few first-hand studies of reaction against cultural disintegration. The typical picture in the third quarter of the twentieth century is that of a wholesale abandonment of time-honoured taboos, especially as regards sexual behaviour. Those whom cultural disintegration brings nearest the brink of personal disaster recoil most vehemently therefrom. To the more earnest thinking members of a younger generation who have had bitter experience of the effects of drink and sexual laxity in the older, the uncompromising discipline of the Mormons or of other neo-Puritan movements proves attractive.

Margaret's father had borne the brunt of cultural disintegration within his family. His father had committed suicide; subsequently his mother had had a baby that could not have been her husband's. His two sisters were women of easy virtue. He himself became obsessed with the idea that the whole world was evil, and determined to protect his own family from temptation. His wife was afraid to dress smartly, was never allowed out unless she took her children with her, and if she was not back by 10 p.m. he went to look for her. To be able to go to a bingo session she had to invent the excuse of visiting her aunt. She had deserted temporarily on at least three occasions. Although there may not have been wordy or violent quarrelling in such an authoritarian family, the basic cause of insecurity – marital disharmony leading to a danger of loss of the mother – was present, as in the more standard type of pattern A.

Conditioned by terror against demonstrative nuisance, Margaret became as obsessional a thief as her father was obsessionally virtuous. She would steal from the teacher's desk in front of all the class while the teacher went to the door, reckoning that none would tell out of fear. After each theft she was very contrite, but stole again. She stole from people from whom she sought affection, notably from an aunt of whom she was fond. It seemed a case of genuine compulsion: owing to the unreliability of her mother as a parent she could not afford openly to reject her father, so her resentment against him had to express itself in an unconscious form. In school she was an inhibited, depressed child.

George's mother was described as well-nigh mentally deficient. The father kept away from the home as much as he could, but had no compunction about bringing two of his illegitimate children back to his wife to look after, and she just accepted them. The marital quarrels centred on the mother's financial ineptitude. George showed a typical pattern of hostility in the home, being moodily rejecting and defiant. He had run away many times and stayed out very late despite punishment. His teachers never had an opportunity to get to know him since he persistently refused to go to school. When pressure was applied and attempts were made to accompany him the short distance, he would get up early and leave the house. He was never a good mixer with other children and always truanted by himself. Moreover, the father blamed him for the family troubles and threatened to have him put away. The mother accused the father of being harsh, whereas he accused her of spoiling the boy. The child's situation seemed a combination of the quarrelling and of the black-sheep pattern, further examples of which are met in the following two cases.

The black-sheep pattern

Arthur was a whimpering, tiresome baby, and as a toddler used to wander off and get lost. He had always been enuretic and a head-banger, had a nervous tic, shouted in his sleep, and was subject to powerful fears, especially of the doctor and dentist and of being alone in the dark. In contrast to the families discussed above, his was a respectable churchgoing one. But the father was disgusted with the boy and feared he would have a bad effect on his four other children. Just as the impaired, affectionally unrewarding infant can induce rejection in the mother, in this case the child's unappealing ways had induced his father to reject him. When not in a hostile mood Arthur was impulsive, cheerful, and irrepressible, and had all the signs of inconsequence and over-reaction.

His behaviour in the home afforded an extreme example of hostility, calculated to make it impossible for him to continue living there. He stole from both parents, choosing, besides money, things that it was very inconvenient to lose, and finally raided the gas meter. He had run away twice and truanted persistently. It seemed as if he was determined to meet his father's threats of putting him away with counter-rejection. He openly said that he did not care if this happened to him, and even bragged to this effect before other boys. On the day that he was charged with breaking into a house he stole his father's new suit and his mother's electric iron and pawned them. In the approved school he remained a behaviour problem and could not earn his release.

Frank was also a neurally and physically impaired child, as evidenced by a squint, unnatural head posture, enuresis, and his extreme puniness and paleness. The father had a fixation on his own mother, and deserted his wife to go back to her when the boy was one and a half years old. On his return some five years later the father became antagonistic to Frank and, himself a former athlete, was notably disappointed in the boy's poor physique. Like the father of the previous boy he was afraid that the younger children would become contaminated with Frank's bad ways, and threatened and pretended to turn him out of the house. The boy ran away from the home some five times, once staying away all night. Apart from this he showed none of the usual symptoms of hostility. In school his maladjustment was of the K type, that of unconcern about adult attachments and lack of moral compunction.

A performance-inadequate family

Harry belonged to the type of family aptly characterized by Wilson[79] as 'performance inadequate'. The mother was a poor manager, a heavy smoker, and a frequenter of public houses. She complained that her husband never spent much time at home since he too went out drinking. Neither parent showed much concern for the children, and the family was finally broken up following eviction for non-payment of rent. Except that some semblance of housekeeping was preserved they would have come in pattern C of the slum-breakdown family, but they more nearly resembled H, a pattern of neglect of the children by parents bent on their own indulgences. They were typical representatives of the low-standard, happy-go-lucky group of Jephcott and Carter,[30] encountered at the point where things go wrong and they lapse into the demoralized group. The insecurity and impermanence of such a life in themselves constitute a stressful situation to the children, but in fact the two elder brothers had survived it and were serving in the merchant navy (to gain entry to which a comparatively clean record is needed). Harry suffered the added stress of pattern F: his father never did like him and made the usual threats of having him put away. Once again the reason seems to have been that he was an emotionally unrewarding child. As an infant he never cried when hurt or punished, and was puny and delicate. At home he showed none of the emotional turbulence of hostility. He did not steal provocatively or run away; on the contrary he was described by his mother as of even temperament, but deceitful, and unconcerned about punishment. At school he showed an extreme maladjustment with a score of 52 indications. The K syndrome predominated (13 indications), with some hostility to adults and strong antisocial attitudes to other children. Together with his early defect of attachment need and his physical and neural impairments the relative lack of hostile response is understandable. For there to be resentment at deprivation the love has to be wanted; there would be no incentive to have done with an unreliable relationship if anxiety about it were absent.

Cultural disintegration

Mabel also suffered from the K type of maladjustment (with a record total score of 65). She showed signs of the moral defect of psychopathy, notably in extorting money from younger girls. At home she did not display much feeling, and wanted to go and live with her married sister. The home answered to the C slum-breakdown pattern, with the typical dirt and smell, and lapse of civilized standards. Although living in a 'black spot' the family were shunned by neighbours. The children were underfed, dirty, and poorly clothed, and the mother was always in debt. This pattern adds its distinctive stress in that the children are neglected, do not get regular meals, and lack all the material solicitudes that serve as daily evidence and reassurance of affection. As Wilson points out in her study of fifty-two such families,[79] the essence of the family situation is its undependability. It is important, however, to realize that the demoralization is the result of the mother's having succumbed to other stresses in her family life, most of which originate in the physical or mental ill health of the husband and the consequent poverty. In this instance the father was physically broken down following a serious accident, but he was also a heavy drinker and a violent man, and the parents were known to quarrel. He could not bear the noise of the children in the house and was harsh to them. Under these stresses the mother had fallen into a state of depression and of irritable-depressive non-tolerance towards Mabel, who was the youngest of her five children.

The girl had multiple physical and neural impairments – a squint, restless sleep, nervous mannerisms, 'jumpiness', finger-sucking (at thirteen years), and bad nailbiting, and she also had frequent colds and was very puny. The father's accident had occurred some years previously, and he was in hospital at the time of Mabel's birth, so that the general family situation could not have been very different for the three elder siblings. Her two elder brothers had secured their removal from it, the one by joining the merchant navy, the other the army. They spent their time ashore or on leave with their married sister and not with their parents. Yet they had survived the family stresses during their school years and earlier adolescence without apparent ill effects. Only the vulnerable child succumbed.

Cultural deviance

Cyril's family cherished a cultural tradition strongly at variance with that of the dominant legal culture. They believed in taking the law into their own hands quite literally, by violence. The father was serving a four years' sentence for assault. Hearing that in his absence his wife had taken a boy-friend he threatened her in his letters from prison, underlining what he was going to do to her when he came out. As an interim measure he sent his own mother to administer punishment: while his brothers held his wife the mother beat her, which earned her thirty days' imprisonment.

When the case was brought before the conference the family had for some months been living in terror of the father's homecoming. The mother was under hospital treatment for nervous disorders and diabetes and had understandably fallen into a state of irritable-depressive non-tolerance. She had a fantasy of hearing her doctor tell her, 'Either you kill that boy or he'll kill you'. She was planning to desert the home before her husband's release and take her daughter with her. But she had no plans for Cyril, and came to the Welfare Officer asking for him to be taken off her hands. The boy reacted to the desertion threat by typical hostility, pilfering food and money from his mother and staying out late.

This behaviour, calculated to sever the bond between himself and his mother, showed that what affected him was not so much his father's imprisonment or his threats to his mother as the fear that she, the available parent, proposed to abandon him (pattern J). The imminence of family crisis caused him to resort to delinquent avoidance-excitement. He snatched goods from shops and vans. Once he stole bread and fed some ducks with it; another time he stole potatoes and pelted them. He was a persistent truant, which is unusual at the tender age of 7½. His need for sensory stimulation was such that he would get up at 6 a.m. and go out even in heavy rain, sometimes not returning until late at night.

His mother said that he refused endearments and had been unaffectionate from infancy. His father rejected him and made an open favourite of his sister. Once again we see affectional unresponsiveness as the starting-point of rejection and counter-rejection. At school the boy showed a mixture of hostility and of 'writing off' of adults and their moral standards – the latter to the extent of shameless acts of stealing. He frequently stole from the teacher's cupboard and desk, sometimes from under her nose.

Unstable unions

It is understandable that pattern J – the fear of abandonment – should be found in an unstable union.

Victor's parents were not married, but had lived together on and off for several years. The mother's two elder children were by another man, Victor being the eldest of three by the present 'husband'. The latter said that he had met the mother at a welfare agency, and had taken pity on her and given her a roof. He would periodically desert her and go to live in his old lodgings, leaving her with no money. But he would come back after a short while, notably when he was out of work and the family became an economic asset, only to desert again when he restarted. She always accepted him back. Occasionally he would decide that she was a nuisance and tell her to clear out, whereupon she would get temporary lodgings in a near-by house. There were phases when they were living apart but seeing each other daily. Their life when they were together was punctuated with quarrels and threats to desert.

Considering the insecurity of such a situation Victor gave evidence of surprisingly little hostility or anxiety. The father showed a constant concern for him, coming to inquire about him at school even when he was not living with the mother. The Welfare Officer reported that he had beautiful toys stored in a cupboard to give the children at Christmas. It seems that a family situation such as this – or the previous one, fraught with violence – which horrifies decent-living people (i.e. those who subscribe to the conventional mores), is not necessarily emotionally intolerable to the child provided there is one reliable parent. Apparently Victor's father, who gave evidence of his affection and never vanished from the scene completely, met this criterion in some degree.

The boy's behaviour disturbance was of the inconsequential sort. He was too restless to remember correction for long, followed other children in mischief and foolish pranks, and took the initiative in rough, boisterous play. With a gang he broke into railway property and was once convicted of larceny. Possibly his inability to give his attention to anything for more than a fleeting moment saved him from taking his family troubles too seriously.

Loss of surrogate parent

Edward's mother was also a cultural deviant. By different men with whom she had cohabited she had had eight children. The grandmother, with whom the family lived, was suspected of keeping a disorderly house and the children were supervised by a child-protection agency owing to their flea-bitten and poorly clad condition. Some five years earlier, when the mother went away for a period to a training home, the five children she had at the time, Edward among them, were taken into the care of the local authority and placed in a children's home. He and his younger brother had recently returned to live with his mother when his case was brought up for consideration. The Welfare Officer and the Health Visitor agreed that the mother was now caring for her family well and seemed fond of them. She was living with an even-tempered man in regular work who would have married her had he been able to get his own wife to divorce him. For no reason that could be discovered, Edward resented this man's presence in the home, pointing out tearfully to the Welfare Officer that he was not his father nor married to his mother. On the other hand, he was keen to talk about the superintendent of the institution and his wife, although he did not want to return there. He seemed all at sea as to which to make his attachment group: his former institution, or his home which had been invaded by a stranger. In the following months, while remaining exemplary at school, his conduct at home deteriorated into a regular pattern of extreme hostility. He damaged furniture and his clothing, stole money from a prepayment television, did not come home for his meals, and once stayed out all night without saying where he had been. He truanted persistently, nonchalantly ignoring the advice and admonishments of welfare workers, magistrates, and police, and was finally sent to an approved school. It was quite evident that he wanted, consciously or otherwise, to secure his removal from a home where he felt ill at ease and unwanted. Being a generally well-adjusted boy – his school rating put him in the 'stable' category – he achieved his purpose by truancy, the least antisocial behaviour needed to secure his committal. His only delinquency was that, with a Jewish boy, he made house-to-house collections in aid of 'Trees for Israel'.

Kenneth also reacted by hostility to being deprived of a surrogate parent. He was one of illegitimate twins who had spent their earlier childhood with their mother and the maternal grandfather. The latter favoured Kenneth as the boy, would not let his mother punish him, and brought him home presents while ignoring his twin sister. When the twins were just over seven years old the mother was able to get a house on her own and leave the grandfather. Nevertheless he continued his favouritism, going to the school to give the boy sweets but giving none to the girl. About a year later he died. This marked the onset of behaviour disturbance in the boy, and he was referred to a child guidance clinic. The mother had always resented the grandfather's interference, and the boy must have seen her as a hard person who was denying him the good things that the loving grandfather wanted to give him. He ran away from home and showed other symptoms of hostility.

In school he combined hostility and attention-seeking with extreme inconsequential over-reactivity. Besides all the usual elements of the latter pattern he threw stones at a teacher in the street and used bad language to other teachers on public buses. He was constantly involved in fights at school. In his case the inconsequence and over-reactivity could be directly related to brain damage. From the age of eleven he began to have epileptic fits and was eventually sent to an epileptic colony, but more because of his violent behaviour than the fits. He also had a speech defect and other somatic and neural impairments. During the pregnancy the mother must have suffered considerable emotional distress. Her own mother had died a little time previously, and since she did not get on well with her father she left home in the fifth month of the pregnancy without telling him, and entered a hostel for unmarried mothers. There she remained, with her brother acting as a go-between, until she returned home with the twins a little time after they were born.

Marilyn was the third of the difficult trio of girls who figured in the earlier part of this series. Like the two boys described above she resented separation from a surrogate parent, in her case a spoiling paternal grandmother. The mother would not let her visit the latter because she disapproved of the happy-go-lucky standards of her home. When, owing to the tactful intervention of the School Welfare Officer, the mother relaxed the ban, the girl showed a marked improvement and began to concentrate upon her work.

The return to the real mother from a surrogate parent is a frequent but little suspected cause of maladjustment, and it is typical that there were no fewer than four instances in this series.

Sidney, who makes the fourth, lost his mother when only a few months old and was reared by his grandmother and an aunt. His father rarely visited him, but took him into his home when he remarried. His step-mother was extremely good with him, but he refused to accept her and, following a quarrel in the house, knocked her down in the street and fled to his aunt. He ran away from home no fewer than five times in all, and showed the usual symptoms of provocative hostility.

Nevertheless, as in many of the other cases described, this behaviour was not simply a matter of response to a depriving situation. Even before Sidney was taken from his grandmother he was on probation for theft, and had been sexually assaulted by an elderly man. It is seldom in such situations that the alleged victim is wholly guiltless. Later, when staying with his aunt, he was a trial to her also: he spoilt a newly decorated room by knocking a hole in the wall, stole cigar-ettes, and ran up an account at a shop at which she dealt.

At school, apart from a certain amount of attention-seeking, he showed little general maladjustment. Other boys called him by a girl's name because of his effeminate appearance, his peculiar walk, and his high-pitched voice. Caught stealing at school also, he was put on probation a second time. His surreptitious and fraudulent thefts from those around him suggested a fundamental impairment of the attachment needs. He had fits which were thought to be epileptic, and was enuretic and pigeon-toed. Unfortunately, with the research resources available, it was not possible to investigate further the reason for the mother's death or whether she was ill during the pregnancy. The boy's sister, one year older, had also been delinquent.

Family Situation and Type of Maladjustment

In reviewing these cases in which a maladjustment-conducive family situation was recognized, we have to ask, first, whether any regular correspondence emerges between the type of depriving situation and the type of maladjustment. Of the fifteen, six met the criterion* for strong hostility (7 or more indications), and one (with 6 indications) came within the moderate range. The three most hostile – with 10 indications or more – were associated with severe parental quarrelling accompanied by desertion threats (pattern A) and rejection by the father (pattern F). But there were also three very pronounced instances of affectionless character (type K maladjustment) associated with the same patterns. Strong HA and K were often found in the same child, and these two types of maladjustment seemed joint or alternative reactions to acutely insecure and depriving family situations, the particular admixture possibly depending upon individual temperament or other special circumstances. A child could exhibit high hostility in the home as a direct outcome of the unreliability of his situation, yet show unconcern for adult attachments and cold rejection in school. In other cases active hostility was transferred to the teacher. Whether such transfer of attitude takes place may be decided by the reactions of the third party, or even by fortuitous resemblances of face, voice, or gesture which evoke conditioned attitudes.

When one is dealing, as here, with a small number of cases the degree of confidence that can be placed in an observed tendency depends upon whether the exceptions can be explained. There were three cases among the fifteen who showed neither the HA nor the K reaction. Margaret – the girl with the obsessionally strict father – displayed only unforthcomingness and depression. The two younger siblings had attended a child guidance clinic on account of nervous fears. Possibly the rigour of the paternal discipline had conditioned them from an early age against any kind of demonstrative naughti-

* See *The Social Adjustment of Children.*[75]

ness. Margaret's stealing might have been an unconscious form of hostility. Victor was an exception only in that the HA and K were rated, with 4 and 5 indications respectively, in the 'some' rather than the 'strong' category. He was an extremely inconsequential boy with a 'restlessness' score of 10. If inconsequence is due to a type of neural impairment that makes conditioning difficult there may also be more resistance to conditioning towards hostility in a depriving situation. The threats of putting away would 'go in one ear and out the other', and the child – having no capacity for temporal integration – would live in a world of immediacy in which a general situation would be forgotten. The last exception, Edward, had spent some years in an institution and gave the impression, so far as his mother and his teachers were concerned, of relative non-involvement, although he did show some hostility to his mother. These exceptions are thus seen to be more apparent than real, and a general relationship seems to emerge between a contemporary security-depriving family situation and the hostile (HA) and rejecting (K) types of maladjustment.

Impaired as well as Deprived

The second general observation to be made from a study of this last group of cases is that somatic and neural impairments were just as prevalent among them as among the two earlier groups. Only two of the fifteen children were free of any such symptoms, and where impairment occurred it tended to be multiple. One also had the impression that the impairment extended to the neural structures which are the seat of behaviour. In particular, whether the child reacted by hostility or not seemed to depend upon the intactness of the attachment need.

Table 3 Fifteen children in critically stressful family situations

Name	*Age*	*BSAG score*	*Delinquency*	*No. of siblings*	*Behaviour of siblings*	*Family situation*	*Type of maladjustment**	*Somatic and neural impairment*	*Congenital factors*
Desmond	14	38	1 serious	7	All stable	A	HA 13 XA 15	Black-outs, dizzy turns; restless sleep; enuresis	
Samuel	13	58	Persistent	7	Unstable delinquent	A	HA 12 K 9 XC 7 D 7	Headaches	
Jean	14	31	None	2	Stable	A	K 11	Restless sleep	
Margaret	12	26	Persistent	3	Unstable	A variant	U 6 D 5		
George	11	(School refuser)	None	3	Stable	A+F		Watery eyes	Forced marriage in late pregnancy
Arthur	12	45	Persistent	4	1 minor delinquent	F	HA 10 D 8	Whimpering, delicate as baby; wanderer, tiresome as toddler; speech defect, nervous tic; enuresis, very disturbed sleep	
Frank	13	29	None	3	Unstable	F	K 9	Squint; enuresis; very pale and puny; unnatural posture of head	

Harry	14	52	Minor	5	Stable	F+H	K HA	13 7	Did not cry as baby; frequent colds and headaches; restless sleep	
Mabel	13	65	Persistent	4	Stable	A+C	K HA XA R	9 8 8 9	Squint; very puny; skin troubles; 'jumpy', nervous mannerisms; restless sleep; bad nailbiter	Father had serious accident during the pregnancy or just previously
Cyril	7½	32	Persistent	1	Stable	G+J	K HA	7 6	Unaffectionate as young child; unclear speech; 'jumpy'	Mother diabetic
Victor	14	30	Persistent	2 full 2 step	Stable? delinquent and m.d.	J	R	10	Athetoid hand movements; bad nailbiter	Illegitimate; unstable cohabitation of parents
Edward	13	4	Minor	7	Stable	I			Restless sleep	Illegitimate; temporary cohabitations of mother
Kenneth	13	37	Minor	1	Stable	I	HA XA	8 7	Epilepsy; speech defect; suspect stomach ulcer; restless sleep; headaches; nosebleeding; bad nailbiter	Illegitimate in distressing circumstances; mother in hostel from fifth month of pregnancy
Marilyn	13	18	None	1	Stable	I				
Sidney	14	10	Persistent	1 full 2 half	Unstable Stable	I			Epilepsy; enuresis; homosexual (?); pigeon-toed; unnatural posture	Mother died when boy was a few months old

* See Appendix II

CHAPTER FOUR

General Conclusions from the Case Studies

Implications for the Causation of Maladjustment

In nearly half of this sample of thirty-three cases at least one of the standard maladjustment-conducive family situations was identified, and in almost as many there existed a degree of stress that might be accounted an aggravating factor. In only two was there early deprivation, and in both it took the form of transfer from the true to a surrogate mother. There were, however, five children who had been reared in stable families without apparent emotional deprivation. In these cases there was positive evidence of parental affection and constancy despite the child's disturbed behaviour. The mean maladjustment score for the eighteen children for whom data were available in Groups I and II – that is to say, those subjected to minimal or subcritical stress – was 25·8, compared with 33·9 for the fourteen scored in Group III, the critical-stress group. Owing to the small size of the sample and the wide variation in scores the difference between the means is not significant statistically, but the trend is consistent with the general view that maladjustment is related to familial stress. That the difference was not greater makes it reasonable to conclude that adverse family situation is an important but not the only factor.

A syndrome of somatic-neural impairment

More striking because hitherto less taken account of was the high incidence of somatic-neural impairment, affecting no fewer than twenty-eight of the thirty-three cases. In six there was diagnosed or suspected epilepsy, with which were associated fourteen other symptoms; there were two instances of squint, associated with nine other symptoms; and nine of defective speech, occurring with twenty-one other symptoms. If enuresis and restless sleep are counted as one symptom when they occurred together, and early behaviour disturbance such as nuisance or wandering is ignored, the fourteen children who had one or more of the epilepsy-squint-speech group showed thirty-eight other symptoms, giving an average of 2·7 per child. The nineteen remaining children had a total of twenty-five symptoms, an average of 1·3. The distribution, presented in *Table 4*, gives a X^2 of 6·68 ($n=1$) by a division of the cases above and below the mean, which amounts to a risk of chance of less than 1 in 100. Where, in short, there were symptoms indicating neural damage – which would

Table 4 Grouping of symptoms

	Cases with less than the mean number of other somatic-neural symptoms	*Cases with more than the mean number of other somatic-neural symptoms*	*Total*
Cases with at least one symptom in the epilepsy-squint-speech group	5	10	15
Other cases	14	4	18
Total	19	14	33

for the most part be of congenital origin – there was a significant excess of other somatic-neural impairment. The implication is that a multiplicity of physical susceptibilities and weaknesses, including certain habit disorders such as enuresis and other symptoms classed as psychosomatic, may also have a congenital origin. This does not preclude their being aggravated by postnatal stresses, as indeed sometimes happens with epilepsy, speech defect, and squint. The extremely high incidence of this whole group of conditions among these disturbed children forces us to consider whether behaviour disturbance may in general belong to the same group of disorders – that is to say, has its origin in some type of congenital or other neural impairment, but is aggravated when the affected person is exposed to a stressful situation.

Perusal of the three tables summarizing the case data shows a wide range of diverse symptoms. Among them those indicating neural impairment are preponderant, but even these take many forms. The syndrome is therefore a loose one consisting of a very large number of alternative manifestations. Any one appears only in a minority of the cases. By the law of probability some would appear in isolation, and behaviour disturbance – if it is a component of the syndrome as hypothesized – could sometimes be the sole symptom. Consequently it cannot be assumed that when a maladjusted child shows no other somatic-neural impairment the behaviour disturbance is without any basis in neural damage.

We seem to be left, in short, with two powerful causal factors in maladjustment: on the one hand, adverse upbringing and contemporary family situation; and, on the other, a susceptibility to stress which is likely to be congenital. It cannot be presumed, however, that these factors are independent of each other. The possibility remains that the same general types of stressful family situation, with the physical stress and deprivation that accompany them, may also have been responsible for the neural damage to the children before or at birth. More detailed data upon the children's early development and upon birth and pregnancy complications would have been invaluable for the corroboration of this hypothesis. It was possible to glean only partial information where it was forthcoming in the course of the School Welfare Officer's contact with the mother, or in the few cases where, subsequent to the case conference, the Welfare Officer was able to make direct inquiry. Nevertheless, the plausibility of the above hypothesis can be subjected to a rough test by examining the third group of fifteen cases in which a critically stressful family situation was present. It is seen from the last column of *Table 3* that in seven instances there was some evidence or grounds for presumption that during the pregnancy the mother suffered either physical ill health or severe emotional stress. In three of these – where the mother was cohabiting temporarily with various men (Edward) or intermittently with the same one (Victor), or the unmarried mother-to-be fled from her irate father into a hostel (Kenneth) – the acuteness of the mental stress cannot be questioned. In three of the four other cases in which a pregnancy factor was specifically mentioned it must be taken in conjunction with marital situations very unlikely to have allowed the woman a healthy, happy, well-nourished pregnancy: in one the father avoided the company of his near-feebleminded wife and asked her to accept two illegitimate children by other women

(George); in a second the pattern was that of slum demoralization with quarrelling, desertion threats, and child neglect (Mabel); the third was that of the violent husband who assaulted his wife vicariously from prison (Cyril). In only one case – that of the mother who died when the child was a few months old (Sidney) – were there no grounds for assuming a stressful pregnancy.

If we now turn to the eight cases with no specific entry for a congenital factor we find very much the same picture. In only three were there no grounds for inferring an unhappy or otherwise stressful pregnancy (Marilyn, Arthur, Desmond). Of the remaining five there were two where the husbands would not work and whose families subsisted on National Assistance, with which went quarrels, violence, and desertion threats (Samuel and Jean). In the case of the obsessionally straitlaced husband, the wife must continually have been subjected to frustrating and stressful episodes, and had in fact deserted temporarily several times (Margaret). The fourth was that of the feckless parents who were later evicted for non-payment of rent (Harry); and the fifth was the case of the husband with the mother-fixation who, before deserting, had spent every evening in his mother's house (Frank). Among these fifteen cases there was thus a probability of a stressful pregnancy in twelve. Of the three cases in which there was no evidence to go on, two had signs of somatic-neural impairment, so that they might not have been exceptions had the full facts been available.

The type of family situation that is stressful enough to the child to induce behaviour disturbance is, if these cases are typical, likely also to be stressful to the mother during her pregnancy. Hence no correlation, however strong, between maladjustment and type of family situation justifies an assumption that the maladjustment can be explained entirely in terms of influences that the child experiences subsequent to birth.

The Cultural Aspects of Maladjustment

The concept of maladjustment is essentially one of the failure of an individual to conduct himself in his own best interests or with regard to the wellbeing of those affected by his actions. It covers a wide range, from behaviour that is actively injurious to the doer or his victims, to a lack of behaviour as in withdrawal, depression, unforthcomingness, or 'laziness'. But the characterization of a person's behaviour as maladjusted has to be made in relation to the normal, accepted standards of his social group. The recognition of this fact has led to a tendency to explain away much maladjusted behaviour, especially when of a deviant or delinquent variety, in merely cultural terms. Either it is discounted as really the normal behaviour of a social group, which is viewed as maladjusted by representatives of the dominant culture because it flouts their standards and ideas of right and wrong; or it is seen as the expression of cultural conflict, that is to say, the resentment of the members of a particular subculture against having 'foreign' standards of behaviour imposed upon them.

Intrinsic maladjustment and cultural deviance

We have consequently to discriminate between cultural variations in behaviour and intrinsic disturbance or instability. A failure to use intellectual potentialities would rank more highly as a symptom of maladjustment in the cultural setting of an aspiring middle class than it would within a less demanding traditional working-class culture. For an adult or adolescent to get involved in a fight would similarly be accounted more reprehensible from the standpoint of the middle class. On the other hand, to be individualistic or innocuously non-conforming would be condoned or even admired in the more intellectual middle-class subcultures, but regarded as almost insulting in a military academy or in a pre-industrial tribal community. But these cultural value differences apply to only a segment of social behaviour, and the mistake has been to exaggerate them and to offer them as a general explanation of every kind of behaviour that is disapproved by members of the dominant culture. If, however, a careful compilation were made of all the categories of behaviour condemned by the dominant group, there is no doubt that the greater number would also be condemned by members of all cultures. Injury and nuisance remain such even though they may be tolerated to a greater degree in one social group than in another. The tiresomeness of a child who as a baby screams for several weeks almost without end, who as a toddler wanders off as soon as the mother's back is turned, or who is always clinging and whimpering; the child of school age who annoys neighbours by breaking their windows, who goes missing for hours at a time, who pilfers the housekeeping money, who ill-treats younger brothers or sisters, or who causes anxiety by his foolhardy escapades; the adolescent girl who runs off with a married man, or the adolescent boy who truants from work and steals to provide a substitute for his wages; the husband who idles his days in bed, who spends his wages on drink and is violent to his wife when she remonstrates; the wife who deserts the home in the course of an extramarital affair, or who squanders her housekeeping money on trifles beyond her means – all these sorts of maladjusted behaviour transcend particular subcultural variations. No culture tolerates theft from a member of the in-group. The degree of violence tolerated is small and strictly regulated to disciplinary or ritual (including sporting) occasions. Insulting, provocative, or rude behaviour – which constitutes attack upon another person's sense of personal worth and effectiveness – is everywhere held reprehensible. Anything, in short, that is liable to divide or disintegrate the family or the in-group, or that causes personal stress beyond the limit of normal forbearance, is outlawed within all cultures. These are the sorts of maladjustment that are the subject of this study.

Culture and exposure to stress

The recognition that maladjustment is something more than a cultural artifact does not throw us back upon purely psychological explanations. When the psychologist studies behaviour he does so with the understanding that its evolutionary value has been to enable organisms to achieve a measure of control over their environment, or to move from a less favourable environment to a more favourable one. Behaviour apart from the environment is meaningless. The psychologist also recognizes that one of man's major evolutionary achievements has been his ability to transmit knowledge, skills, customs, values, and successful institutional forms from one generation to another, and such a body of transmitted 'know-how' is called a culture. The type of the culture exercises a decisive influence upon the behaviour of every individual who subscribes to it. It also largely determines his means of livelihood and his standard of life. The survival value of any culture is expressed in its effectiveness in preserving man from the chances and dangers of purely instinctive animal existence. In short, an intact culture, exercised within the ecology where its success has been demonstrated by survival, preserves against stress or, more exactly, reduces stresses to the level at which they no longer jeopardize the existence of the social group.

It is this concept of a tolerable level of stress that forms one important link between sociology and psychology. Beyond a certain point we know that human beings tend to break down either physically or emotionally. Their normal, circumspect pattern of behaviour gives way to a pattern of stress behaviour. If there is a failure of cultural transmission, that is to say, if the culture disintegrates, human behaviour loses its directive framework. Individual desires take precedence over the traditional code which, by and large, has worked for the general good in that it has enabled many generations of a local population to survive and to thrive. Stresses upon other members of the group are consequently multiplied, and the amount of personal breakdown is increased.

Among the most important of human cultural institutions has been that of the family. In the present study we have seen a number of instances where its disintegration or unreliability, from the child's point of view, has produced a stress situation to which the child responded by maladjustment. Thus cultural changes affect the child not only by their direct impact upon him but by the manner in which they influence his family life. If we wish to follow this process in detail we have to trace the origin in cultural terms of the maladjustment-conducive family situations that have been identified. More specifically, we have to ask whether they were the result of inappropriateness of the cultural heritage to contemporary conditions of life; of loss or disintegration of the culture; or of a clash of cultures.

The cultural background to stressful family situations

Since the stressful family patterns were seen at their critical level in the fifteen cases of Group III, they will be taken as the subject of analysis. In five of them the situation was such as might arise in a culturally intact family in harmony with its environment. The difficulties centred on individual weaknesses or calamities – the rejection by the father of a tiresome, neurally impaired child; the mother-fixation of a husband; the trials of an unmarried mother; a wife's illicit affair.

Seven instances – nearly half those under review – were characterized by cultural disintegration or deprivation. Two fathers refused to work; another defied the marital conventions to the extent of planting his illegitimate children on his wife; parents followed a life of feckless pleasure while neglecting their children; other parents reverted to casual mating; a home became demoralized following an accident to the husband. These cases differed from the sexual lapses included in the first group in that they represented a persistent non-observance of the accepted code. The parents were heedless of the sanctions that would have secured the code's enforcement in a closely knit, culturally intact community. In a culture where social discipline is maintained by tribal law or the hegemony of a religious leader, and deviance is checked by the threats of ostracism or curse, there is no great need for the self-discipline of the independent Puritan way of life. The individual indulges his day-to-day desires up to the point where he senses that he may make trouble for himself with fellow-members of his face-to-face group. Strength of character and individual moral rectitude are not subscribed to as abstract ideals. If the members of such hedonistic cultures are wrested from their social framework in the tribe or village the restraints are removed without being replaced, as in a migrating middle-class family, by habits of individual discipline. There will be no relatives and neighbours whose opinion matters, and they are no longer under the eye of the priest. In old-established urban communities the traditional pattern can be re-established, as Young and Willmott have shown,[82] but all too often the family will move from one neighbourhood to another within the city, and lose contact with or, if they are tending towards deviance, be avoided by, their kith and kin. Wilson[79] found it to be characteristic of her performance-inadequate families that they were thus isolated. The isolation also means that the network of mutual obligation upon which the hedonistic family depends for help in times of adversity is no longer in existence. As Wilson emphasizes, the condition of such families does not constitute a specific subculture, but a breakdown of culture; she adds that 'these socially isolated families are in danger of regressing to the animal level of survival with all the losses in terms of security and thwarting of individual development that this entails'. Spinley[54] also drew attention to the frequency of maladjustment-producing family situations in an underprivileged urban neighbourhood: 'The child of this city slum is exposed to so many textbook causes of maldevelopment that the problem is not so much why he displays the signs of disturbance which he does, but rather how he manages to continue as a functioning personality. . . .' She described the types of family disintegration or near-disintegration – parental quarrels with violence, 'the coming and going of father or series of fathers', etc. – that were exemplified in the present cases. In their 'Radby' study, Jephcott and Carter[30] point out that the happy-go-lucky family who live for the present can manage provided they meet no calamity in the form of accident or illness. One might add, provided no individual behaves in a way that undermines the economy of the household or indulges his sexual desires in a way that breaks up the family. The present cases afford instances of collapse under such conditions, bringing out in particular the extent to which deviant personality can be a hazard.

Apart from the seven cases that were characterized by cultural disintegration or deprivation, there was one interesting example – in the obsessionally strict father – of reaction against cultural disintegration. In addition, two of the cases studied might be put under a broad heading of cultural conflict. In one, the husband's ideas as to the best means of punishing his wife for her unfaithfulness were at variance with the legal provisions of the dominant culture: he resorted to direct-action methods that would have been judged his right in mediaeval times or in many pre-industrial communities. In the second case the cultural conflict was between two branches of a family, the mother disapproving of the happy-go-lucky, slatternly mode of life of her husband's relatives. It was unfortunate that her daughter, possibly attracted by the spontaneous warmth of personal relationships found in the latter type of culture, developed a primary attachment for a grandmother on the wrong side of the wall.

It must be emphasized that none of the above cases, in which there were cultural factors underlying the pathological family situation, could be characterized as purely 'cultural'. Whether an individual reacts one way or another to cultural stresses depends upon his individual temperament. And the manner in which cultural stresses bear upon people's minds and influence their actions is within the field of psychology. It is unrealistic to attempt to separate cultural from psychological deviance, for each is but a different aspect of a complicated chain of cause and effect, in which processes traditionally regarded as within the realm of sociology and psychology have their part. Both the father who tried to impose a puritanical mode of life on his family and the one who resorted to primitive methods of enforcing his marital rights were personality deviants who, nonetheless, dealt with family situations in the light of their respective cultural backgrounds.

It is not even possible to discount a cultural factor in the first five cases discussed where the pathological situation had no immediate background of cultural stress. When we ask why a tiresome, neurally damaged child should appear in a given family, or why a husband should be mother-fixated, we are thrown into the little-explored field of the interaction between congenital trauma and pregnancy/birth complication. It was found by Drillien[15] that the birth weight and viability of a child are related more closely to the occupation group of the maternal grandfather than to that of the husband; the mother's own physical constitution and childhood conditions counted more than her contemporary economic status. It may be that, as in animal populations, congenital weaknesses arising from environmental stress are transmitted from one generation to another, an impairment in one inducing an impairment of possibly quite a different type in the next. The health and viability of any population, whether animal or human, may well be affected by conditions of life reaching back three or four generations.

CHAPTER FIVE

Pointers to Treatment

Vulnerability

If we can assume that these thirty-three children exemplify the problem of behaviour disturbance within our city schools they will serve as a basis for a consideration of treatment and remedies. Any expectation of wholesale and spectacular cure will be dispelled when it is realized that a good proportion of them were certainly neurally impaired; to judge by the criterion of the presence of other kinds of impairment, probably as many as 80 per cent of the sample could be so described. To make the most parsimonious generalization, they were nearly all temperamentally 'vulnerable' children.

In some the impairment seemed to consist in a defect in the attachment needs and hence in the instinctive feeling for what made them socially acceptable; by their violation of the canons of social behaviour they created stressful situations against themselves. Others were vulnerable in the sense that they were over-sensitized to stress: they had low powers of resistance, or, not being able to inhibit mildly unfavourable elements in their life situations, became over-reactors. A third type of vulnerability was seen in the inconsequential group, who needed to be protected from provoking situations. There was of course an overlap, many of the children being vulnerable in more than one respect.

'Bad stock'

To many social workers the idea that a disturbed child may be congenitally impaired is repugnant because of the pessimism it would seem to imply. But a reaction of this kind suggests a total misunderstanding of the concept, arising partly from a confusion between the terms 'congenital' and 'hereditary'. 'Congenital' means simply that the condition, to quote the *Faber Medical Dictionary*, was 'actually or potentially present at birth'. It could have arisen at the birth itself or during the pregnancy. It includes genetic determination, but the overwhelming body of research evidence suggests that the latter is in the nature of a *potentiality* to a defect or weakness. The impairment usually manifests itself only in the event of prenatal stress,[63] and every individual animal and human being apparently carries an array of the genes for such potential weaknesses. We cannot point to our fellow human beings, even though they be members of multigeneration problem families, and declare that they come of 'bad stock'. Our own stock would probably have produced an analogous crop of defects and weaknesses if it had been exposed to similar stresses. In a practical sense, therefore, we cannot write off a case of behaviour disturbance as being hereditary, even though a congenital basis is suspected. Nevertheless, various substrains within each species have been found to bear genetic potentialities for particular defects. The white race, for example, is especially prone to cleft palate. Many studies of mental illness in identical twins have shown that various psychoses have a genetic basis (this showing itself more consistently in twins because they share the same pregnancy and in addition are a source of prenatal stress to each other).

As regards the potentiality for less severe forms of behaviour disturbance, the most reasonable assumption is that the position is similar to that for common non-epidemic diseases. Although a slight hereditary tendency has been discerned for nearly all of these, whether the individual succumbs or not depends in large part upon his environment and in particular upon the infections to which he is exposed. Because proneness to bronchitis or tuberculosis has a genetic basis no one would insist that these conditions are untreatable. The first prerequisite of therapy is to protect the patient against those stresses that are likely to bring on the disease.

Situational treatment

We can apply exactly the same principle to the treatment of behaviour disturbance: we must try to arrange the situation so that the stresses that are liable to activate the disturbance are kept to a minimum. Since the disturbed person, as has been seen, is liable to involve himself in stressful situations, therapy includes personal guidance and in some cases more thoroughgoing treatment. The main emphasis, however, must be on the easing of the situation, without which individual treatment is carried out against unnecessarily heavy odds. In any case the number of disturbed children is so large that individual treatment other than guidance is out of the question for the great majority.

Impairment need not be permanent

The second reason for the reluctance to accept a congenital factor in maladjustment is the notion that what is congenital is fixed for all time. This is true for malformation of the bodily structure, but not necessarily for neural impairment. It is not at all certain what form the latter takes, and it may not involve actual destruction of cerebral tissue. Even when it does, as in brain injury, other neural structures may take over the functions of the damaged tissue. Humphrey and Zangwill[28] report a case of pronounced defects in the higher visual functions, including dreaming, as a result of a shell wound. Five years later the patient's ability to dream returned, and his powers of visualization also improved greatly.

Impairment may be due to nothing more than a disturbance of the normal sequence of maturation. This explanation seems to apply particularly to cases of inconsequential behaviour. Young children are inconsequential by adult standards, and the inconsequence of persistent adult criminals so resembles the natural behaviour of a young child in this respect that Roper[49] considered their most characteristic personality defect to be emotional immaturity. Hugh, the inconsequential boy who was rescued from the canal, was still a finger-sucker at ten years. With the disturbed girls there seemed to be a tendency for puberty to be delayed, and many of the boys at thirteen and fourteen were notably small for their age. Some were described as 'nice wee boys', with the innocent charm and temperamental resilience of younger children which often enabled them to escape retribution for their misdeeds. It may one day be possible to identify a general delayed-maturation syndrome covering both physical and behavioural development. In *Man Meets Dog* Lorenz[36] remarks how, up to the age of six months, young husky dogs in Eskimo camps are quite incapable of being conditioned to respect the territory of each team, continually marauding and being chased off; but once the critical age is passed they learn straight away. The behavioural propensities of the animal are adapted not only to the needs of the species in general but to those of the young at each stage of their growth. Some kinds of temperamental impairment in human beings could be due to the upsetting of such sequences of maturation.

Prognosis for the impaired

Whether the temperamental impairment is due to tissue damage or delayed maturation there is undoubtedly a tendency to spontaneous correction. This occurs at a slow but steady rate during childhood, and often with dramatic speed following puberty. The writer has known many unforthcoming boys who lacked the confidence to tackle reading in their prepubertal years but who developed normal assertiveness and became educable during adolescence. It is also not unusual for an 'affectionless character', who appears to have no sense of human decency or need for social attachments, suddenly to develop a great fondness for his family in early adolescence; the affectionate side of his nature seems to 'wake up'. The most inconsequential and over-reacting boy the writer has ever known – a case of placenta praevia – whose whole school life consisted in provocation, retaliation, and tears, developed into a sensible young man thanks to being a member of a stable family and of a small club for mentally and emotionally handicapped children. This tendency to grow out of congenital temperamental weakness has many counterparts in physical handicaps. It is seen, especially among boys, in bronchitis, asthma, and defective motor coordination.

Nevertheless, such spontaneous improvement can occur only if the temperamentally impaired child is protected against the stresses to which he is vulnerable. Once the tolerance limit is passed typical stress reactions come into play – temper tantrums or violent impulsive outbursts, irrational removal urges, near-psychotic avoidance compulsions, hostility. The stages of these 'maladjusted' reactions and the rejection and retribution that they provoke succeed each other in a vicious circle. The great majority of our persistent criminals must have been made in this way. It follows that the chief therapeutic objective with the temperamentally damaged child must be that of a holding operation – a playing for time until the processes of maturation have in a measure caught up. The technique consists in removing every source of stress, so far as is practicable, from the child's life, and having someone at hand to deal with crises when they occur so that other people can be persuaded to exercise forbearance. With the parents the tactful explanation that the child is suffering from some nervous trouble which he must be helped to grow out of may convert rejection into tolerance. No type of disturbed child is more in need of oversight and guidance, or responds more thereto, than the congenitally damaged.

The subsequent histories of our particular children will now be reviewed in order to assess the effects of the work of the School Welfare Officers with the facilities for treatment at their disposal.

How the Cases Responded

Group I

Of the five children in Group I – those in stable family situations – three were so temperamentally impaired that it was clearly a matter of holding operations (Hugh, Leslie, Alec). In the sense that none of the three appeared in court and that their behaviour became tolerable these may be accounted successful. With Alec this was only formally true: to his other thefts he added that of stealing the potatoes his mother sent him to buy and pocketing the money. But his form of handicap was a defect of attachment need and consequently a complete lack of guilt. At school he was described as, 'Still a crook, but a more pleasant one than before'. Despite the discovery of his frauds he was never charged in court; people could not understand why such a nice boy should do such things. During the year after he left school he worked in a shop without reported incident. Of the two remaining cases, Malcolm, who combined inconsequence with 'laziness', made no more trouble for himself and worked for a year as a roundsman's boy. The fifth, Janet, was one of the troublesome trio of girls, the handling of whom must be registered to the credit of the School Welfare Officer, since they all settled down well and ceased to be a nuisance. This success was achieved by frequent informal talks with the girls and by an understanding with their teachers that they should allow the Welfare Officer to deal with any flare-up.

Group II: Successful holding operations

Among the thirteen cases of Group II – those in stressful but not classically maladjustment-producing family situations – there were five over-reacting, more or less inconsequential children who were the subject of successful holding operations. In all cases support was given to the parents in order to encourage tolerance of the temperamental defect and to minimize impatient threats of 'putting away'. Roger was reported by his mother to have improved greatly, and he was responsible for no more incidents in school. Herbert was moved into another class and did notably better with other teachers. A definitive diagnosis of epilepsy was made in respect of Mary at a third hospital. In her last year she took to fighting with other girls and got involved in various difficult situations; it was evident that she would still require some form of close supervision. The situations of Duncan and of Stewart were alleviated in a similar way.

Good response to treatment

Three cases in this group had a positively successful outcome in that the child's behaviour changed markedly for the better as a result of the efforts of the Welfare Officer, without subsequent relapse. One of these was Carol, the second of the troublesome trio. After it had been explained to Andrew's parents that they must desist from their threats to send him back to Malta and the idleness of the threat had been made clear to him, he was reported to have become 'a different boy' at home.

The third case was that of Rose who, during her last six months at school, went through a difficult period in which her over-reactivity became accentuated. She would often be sent to the Welfare Officer by one of the teachers with the remark, 'I'm not having you, you'd better go down to Mrs A'. There is no knowing what would have happened if Mrs A had not been at hand. In one of her last weeks at school there was a scene in which she was so truculent as to be threatened with suspension. The Welfare Officer arranged with the mother for Rose to come and have a talk with her in the school during the evening. This talk lasted two hours, and in the course of it 'We got quite a lot of things sorted out'. The girl remained on good terms with the Welfare Officer for her remaining weeks at school and went periodically to see her during her first year at work. This episode illustrates the value of having a Welfare Officer on the spot who is in a position to deal with a crisis in the development of a disturbed adolescent.

On balance, then, it may be said that in eight of the thirteen cases the Welfare Officers' efforts must be accounted successful considering the temperamental instability of the children concerned.

Those who did not respond

Of the remaining five, four were committed to approved schools and one was placed on probation and received twenty-eight days' detention for housebreaking. These developments do not necessarily imply failure of the treatment of the boys concerned from a long-term point of view: it is rather a question of whether any better course might have been found. Among those committed were the two avoidance-compulsion cases: Stanley, whose younger brother was killed outside his house, and Neil, who was left affectionally destitute when his mother died of cancer, required more expert psychological treatment than could be given. Both had been committing hectic delinquent acts and had been subject to irrational impulses for some years, and the nature of their disturbance should have been diagnosed earlier. The symptoms of avoidance compulsion are unmistakable to anyone on the look-out for them. (See 'avoidance-excitement' in *Delinquency and Human Nature*.[55]) A feature of these cases is that they are usually resistant to treatment within their own environment and to punishment, and the children concerned should first be removed from the surroundings that evoke the memory of the emotional trauma. Since their delinquency is unconsciously motivated there can be no justification for any form of committal that has an element of punishment or retribution. At the same time, residential schools where treatment should be undertaken would need the staff complement of an approved school, with the addition of a specialist in maladjustment. Unfortunately neither the schools nor qualified psychologists exist in sufficient quantities to fill this need at present.

Albert and Bernard should also have been removed at an earlier age from their family environments. For the first, the quarrelsome pattern of the family life was too much for his low stress-tolerance and over-reactivity. His history of convulsions in infancy, choroid movements, and early behaviour disturbance should have been an indication for skilled psychiatric guidance. It is hard to think of anything less appropriate for this brain-damaged boy than the twenty-eight days of detention that he was awarded. The fate of Bernard of the family of garbage rummagers, with his three delinquent elder brothers, might also have been predicted and possibly forestalled by residential schooling.

There remains the case of Geoffrey who, although he showed a hankering after escape in his vain efforts to join the navy or the army, did not have a markedly adverse home situation. It was just that his tiresome and feckless behaviour had exceeded his mother's patience, and with his over-sensitivity he could not tolerate the resulting rejection threats. After leaving school he held a job as a van boy for some months, but during a spell of unemployment started to gamble and, evidently falling in with a bad set, resumed his delinquencies. He lived on a rehousing development that had a bad reputation for adolescent misbehaviour but was without any kind of recreational amenities. The evening clubs attached to the schools made attendance at some kind of organized activity, such as physical education or carpentry, compulsory, a regulation that either discourages the more unsettled type of youth or secures his early expulsion. The Mormon church had started an informal gramophone-record club, which was discontinued following objections to Sunday dancing. After that there was not even a café in the neighbourhood to which the local youth could repair, or a shopping centre in which they could legitimately saunter. Meanwhile, as a result of the prevalent misbehaviour, the police carried out antiloitering sweeps, even charging boys who were leaning against the entrances to their own tenement stairs. The Welfare Officer described conditions as 'almost a Mafeking-siege atmosphere', which was generating widespread resentment. If boys like Geoffrey are to have a chance of growing up with the right attitudes to society they need the availability of adults whom they respect and accept during the susceptible years between school-leaving and adulthood. It is suggested in the following chapter (p. 91) that such guidance can be best provided in small, informal clubs.

Group III: Success despite difficult family situations

In Group III, which consisted of the fifteen children judged to be in breakdown-conducive family situations, it could not be expected that the success rate would be as high. Nevertheless, five of them, as a direct result of the efforts of the School Welfare Officers, finished their school careers and survived a year in the outside world without committing further delinquency or nuisance. One was the leader of the difficult trio of girls, Marilyn, who voluntarily stayed on at school six months past the statutory leaving age. Margaret, who showed her unconscious hostility against her obsessionally strict father, was removed to an all-girls' school, following which there were no further outbreaks of stealing. The father was also persuaded to allow his family more latitude. Jean, whose attachment needs seemed defective in her earlier girlhood, sought the guidance of her Welfare Officer about her employment, and kept in touch with her. Whether or not it was because of the contact of the latter with the home it is difficult to say, but just about the time the girl was due to leave school the work-shy father took a job.

The case of Desmond further demonstrates the continued value of the School Welfare Service to children with this kind of background during their first years in employment. On leaving school he got a job with the street-trading firm where his father was employed, and when several pounds of the takings were missing he was unjustly accused of embezzling it. His indignant reply was, 'I certainly knock off something for a packet of fags, but not all that much!' He was a great help to his mother in the house, and when he worked late with his father would see the latter home in a taxi on the occasions when he over-indulged. He would 'phone the Welfare Officer occasionally 'just to let you know I'm alive'. Despite his wish to go to a residential school he never succeeded in getting to one, and after leaving school he was hoping to join the army. One feels that some means ought to have been at hand for relieving a loyal boy of the burden of his family troubles by taking him out of the home.

Frank was the fifth positive success; despite his evident neural impairment and a harassing home situation his pilfering and running away ceased and he worked for a year without incident.

Two other cases had a happy outcome as a result of sensible steps taken by the children themselves to escape from insecure family situations. After his family were evicted for non-payment of rent Harry stayed with a neighbour for a while and was then able to join the merchant navy like his brothers. Mabel, the member of a demoralized slum family, with a record score of sixty-five indications of maladjustment, and multiple indications of somatic-neural impairment, faced a crisis when her mother deserted the home and went to live with another man. While her mother was absent Mabel took upon herself the job of looking after another family of young children whose mother was away. Finally she settled with her aunt, worked regularly at a job, and helped with the aunt's children. With many cases in the writer's experience children and young people in difficult family situations have first explored sensible means of escape before resorting to delinquent acts in order to secure their removal. These two were lucky in being able to find the means of doing so.

Cases for preventive removal

In three other cases no delinquency or other behavioural deterioration had occurred, but it could not be said that a satisfactory solution had been achieved. With his extreme maladjustment and a home situation characterized by an idling and wife-assaulting father and a periodically deserting mother, Samuel was an obvious case for preventive removal. The same could be said of Victor, whose mother later broke off her intermittent cohabitation with the man who found a use for her only as a means of supplementing his National Assistance when unemployed. Sidney, the epileptic, spastic, suspected homosexual who knocked down his stepmother, was taken into the home of one of his mother's sisters, but he could be endured for only a few months; at the time of writing another maternal aunt is looking after him. It is anybody's guess whether these three boys will be able to avoid breakdown for much longer. The obvious indication – the provision of residential accommodation with experienced and expert supervision – could not be followed because no such facilities exist except for those who qualify by persistent delinquency.

Those who secured removal

The remaining five boys were removed from home. George, the school refuser, whose father had brought two illegitimate children for his mentally weak wife to take care of, and Cyril, whose mother fled from the home in anticipation of the release of her vengeful husband from prison, were taken into the care of the local authority. Kenneth was removed to a colony allegedly on account of his epilepsy but really because of his violence. Edward, who found it difficult to accept his mother on his return from a children's home, was sent to an approved school for truancy; and the same fate befell Arthur on account of his housebreaking. With his behaviour disturbance dating back from infancy he had been rejected by his family as the black sheep, and he could not tolerate threats of being put away. His offences were probably committed in moods of hostility when he invited removal, and he admitted that he did not care if this happened. It was the familiar story of the boy who, with a low level of stress-tolerance, finds his situation in the home unbearable, with no means of escape except delinquency. The obvious preventive therapy is to provide a means of escape in the form of a voluntary residential school or industrial training course to which young people in this predicament can go without first qualifying by delinquency. Among the 102 senior approved school boys studied by the writer[55] there was evidence that for fifty-five of them the need to escape formed at least part of the motivation of their delinquency. It follows that if such places could be provided the amount of delinquency would be appreciably reduced.

CHAPTER SIX

Remedies

The Strategy

A school welfare service

The crux of treatment, as has been pleaded in the foregoing chapters, is to discover and to help the emotionally handicapped child before he creates personal and social rejection of himself in a vicious circle. Once this has happened, the child may respond by intractable anti-social and delinquent attitudes.

We need, consequently, to develop a mental health service for children and young people with its main emphasis on prevention. As a result of his experience of children from underprivileged neighbourhoods in Liverpool, J. B. Mays made the following proposal:*

> 'More attention could be given to the possibility of the appointment of trained social workers to the staffs of schools in problem areas to undertake work with families found to be in need of advice and help.
>
> Such workers would be entrusted with the highly responsible and difficult task of maintaining the closest possible link between the schools and home. . . . This task would involve something more constructive than mere liaison and the establishment of support between the teachers and the parents. It would entail positive direction in matters of child care, giving insight to parents regarding the vital phases of child development and the crucial significance of interpersonal relationships in the home. Along with advice and sympathy would go a gentle but firm pressure tending in the direction of more consistent discipline, greater masculine participation in homemaking and wiser household expenditure.'

* *The Times Educational Supplement*, 24 November 1961.

In September 1944 – some seventeen years earlier – a subcommittee of Glasgow City Education Committee, in a report on juvenile delinquency, had come to a similar conclusion, recommending that: 'Specially trained Welfare Officers would appear to have a place in the modern school and the subcommittee are anxious that an experiment in this direction should be made.' This recommendation was accepted by the Education Committee and in the following year three School Welfare Officers were appointed to three secondary schools, two of them from the teaching profession and one a qualified social worker. The service lapsed after three years owing to the return of the teachers to teaching and the emigration of the social worker. An evaluation of the effects of this work on school attendance and delinquency is given in the Third Statistical Account of Scotland,[13] as shown in *Table 5.*

Table 5 Evaluation of School Welfare Service in terms of attendance percentages and delinquency totals 1944–47

School	*1944–45*	*1945–46*	*1946–47*
ATTENDANCE PERCENTAGE			
A	80·5	83·8	86·9
B	81·0	86·0	87·6
C	82·3	86·9	87·4
All Glasgow average	85·4	87·3	88·3
DELINQUENCY TOTALS*			
A	37	33	11
B	65	52	24
C	46	45	30
All Glasgow totals (ages 8–16 years)	2,266	2,540	2,406

Source: Cunnison and Gilfillan (1951)[13]

* Crimes only – roughly corresponding to the English category of indictable offences

It is seen that, at the beginning of the three-year period, attendance rates in the three schools were significantly lower than in Glasgow schools as a whole, but by its end they had nearly reached the average. The delinquency total for the three schools together was more than halved over the period (dropping from 148 to 65 court appearances), whereas that for all Glasgow children rose by some 6 per cent. In view of this encouraging result the service was reinaugurated in 1950 with the appointment of two new officers, and has been progressively augmented until at the present time it comprises seventeen trained social workers and four welfare assistants in attendance at an in-service training course.

An effective policy of prevention requires such a grass-roots service within the schools. Only thus can the vulnerable children, who will otherwise furnish the next generation of criminals and ne'er-do-wells, be reliably discovered. Being within the school itself the Welfare Officer can follow a plan of situational treatment with the minimum disturbance to the child's school or family life. Existing school psychological and child guidance services scarcely touch the fringe of the problem in numerical terms. Their time may be taken up with the ascertainment of mentally retarded children, and a good proportion of children referred for treatment suffer from specific habit disorders and present no general behaviour problem. Attempts to bring parents and children to clinics result in the selection of those cases for treatment in which the parents are cooperative, of normal intelligence, not overburdened with large families, are concerned about the child, and lead comparatively well-organized lives. These criteria would have excluded thirteen or nearly 40 per cent of the present sample of cases. However, the biggest barrier to the effective use of the present psychological services is the failure of schools to refer cases because maladjustment is viewed merely as undisciplined behaviour, wilfulness, or laziness. When a Welfare Officer is at hand in the school, teachers will sometimes mention an incident to her that they describe as merely 'blowing off steam', and yet it may be symptomatic of maladjustment or even brain damage.

A further advantage of a School Welfare Service is that coordination between the various social agencies ceases to present a problem. The Glasgow officers enjoy an informal and harmonious relationship with the probation service, rivalry being obviated for the practical reason that the case loads of the Probation Officers are too large to permit of more than a small amount of the family therapy that might ideally be undertaken. The Welfare Officer is also able, from intimate knowledge of the child's school and home life, to help the Probation Officer in his recommendations to the court.

The opportunity to apply situational treatment as a first line of attack places the Welfare Officer in a position to gauge the point at which more expert psychological help should be called in, or at which the child needs to be removed from his home surroundings. But, as the writer has pointed out,[56] the decision to remove a child from his home can be taken only when it becomes apparent that the child is too disturbed for his family to be expected to tolerate him, or when the family prove resistant to guidance. It has been seen above that the Welfare Officers were able to intervene successfully in several of the present cases even though a state of mutual rejection between parent and child had been reached. The way in which people will respond cannot always be accurately predicted. Unless, therefore, the family situation is seen as obviously deleterious or the child has to be restrained for the safety of those around him, a decision as to his removal should be taken only after a period of family casework. At present, whether or not a child is removed often depends upon fortuitous factors – the nature and number of the offences of which he is found guilty, or the winsomeness of his manner and appearance (one finds few good-looking children in approved schools). True concern both for the welfare of the emotionally handicapped child and for the health of the society that has to bear with him demands a treatment programme based upon the child's needs at any one time. The knowledge that a School Welfare Officer has of a child is invaluable in determining these needs.

A nation-wide service of School Welfare Officers would take time to develop. But throughout Britain many members of the present service of Education Welfare Officers are already carrying out family therapy, incidentally and unofficially, in the course of their school-attendance responsibilities. Their effectiveness is, however, hampered because each officer has to cover a fairly large number of schools and the service lacks the authority and prestige that would be required if it were to be given the main responsibility for the handling of cases. The first step must be to establish courses in the techniques of diagnosis and family casework for, among others, serving Education Welfare Officers, and to secure their recognition as a profession for which in future a full social-work qualification will be needed. Salaries should also be at a level to make feasible the transfer to such a service of teachers who are attracted to the welfare aspects of education.

Since its reconstitution in 1950 the Glasgow School Welfare Service has worked within secondary schools owing to the urgency of the delinquency problem there. Prior to each half-yearly entry of twelve-year-olds from the primary schools the officers visit the latter in order to hear the teachers' views as to which children are likely to present problems at the secondary stage. The result has been that the Welfare Officers have come to be appreciated by primary-school heads, who sometimes seek their help. With the possible exception of the few girls in whom pubertal instability was noted, it can be said with fair confidence that all the children who were the subject of the present study would have been maladjusted in their primary schools. Contrary to the general impression, there is very little variation in the incidence of maladjustment at different ages; it is, if anything, slightly higher among prepubertal children. Among the 598 control children of the truancy survey reported in Chapter Seven, the mean number of indications of behaviour disturbance among children up to their eleventh birthday was 8·23, compared with 7·25 for those aged eleven to fifteen years. A similar slight reduction with age in the severity of maladjustment was found in the controls of Glasgow probationers. Consequently, there is just as great a need for a School Welfare Officer in a primary as in a secondary school. Moreover, a delinquency-prevention service, to be effective, would need to detect the delinquency prone by the eleventh year, since it is most often just after that age that the disturbed child turns to law-breaking.

The incidence of maladjustment among schoolchildren

Official estimates of the incident of maladjustment – amounting to 1 or 2 per cent of the schoolchild population – have been much too low. *Table 6* summarizes the findings of three recent surveys in which the Bristol Social Adjustment Guides were used as the measure of maladjustment:

(i) controls of truants drawn from some hundreds of schools throughout Britain (see Chapter Seven below)
(ii) a carefully randomized sample of Liverpool schoolchildren aged 7 and 8 years (Crawford)
(iii) a sampling of secondary schools in and around Swansea (Chazan[9]).

The data show that between 11 and 15 per cent of boys and 8 per cent of girls are maladjusted in Britain by the criterion of 20 recorded indications of behaviour disturbance. This cut-off point is an arbitrary one, but so that the reader can judge what it means in actual behaviour the items marked for three children scoring 20 or 21 in the truancy survey, but with differing types of disturbance, are listed in Appendix III (p. 193 below). The borderline level of maladjustment shown would seem to come within the definition of the term as employed by the Underwood Committee,* which runs: 'a child may be regarded as maladjusted who is developing in ways that have a bad effect on

* Ministry of Education (1955). *Report of the Committee on Maladjusted Children.* (Chairman: Dr J. E. A. Underwood.) London: HMSO.

himself or his fellows and (whose behaviour) cannot without help be remedied by his parents, teachers and other adults in ordinary contact with him'.

In an average primary school of 500 children there would be some thirty boys and twenty girls at this level or worse, a number that would certainly fully occupy the time of a School Welfare Officer. Their distribution would, however, be very unequal. There would be many more in those schools, both primary and secondary, serving the underprivileged, overcrowded areas of our cities. It is these that should have the first priority for the relatively small number of social workers who can be trained within the next few years.

Table 6 Summary of three surveys of maladjustment in Britain (percentages in each adjustment category)

Sample	Age range in years	N	Score Groups on Bristol Social Adjustment Guides: Stable and quasi-stable (0–9)	Unsettled (10–19)	Maladjusted (20+)
			%	%	%
BOYS					
Controls of truants (Britain)	6–15	429	69·7	19·1	11·2
Random sample (Crawford, Liverpool)	7–8	387	62·4	23·1	14·8
Classes in secondary schools (Chazan, Swansea)		211	61·6	27·5	10·9
GIRLS					
Controls of truants (Britain)	6–15	169	75·7	16·0	8·3
Random sample (Crawford, Liverpool)	7–8	386	72·6	19·7	7·8
Classes in secondary schools (Chazan, Swansea)		211	73·5	19·0	7·6

Three-cornered conferences

Many schools serving more well-to-do areas or in those regions where the traditional culture is intact are unlikely to contain the proportion of maladjusted pupils that would justify the appointment of a full-time officer. This raises the question whether the head can be expected to deal with any difficult cases that do occur. In a smaller school he may have developed a flair for doing so, but it is evident that this is a matter of the interest and talent of the individual head.

While working in the Bristol region the writer, in the course of visits to schools to study causes of retardation, was asked by certain heads for help with troublesome children. It was found that in nearly all cases the mother was prepared to come to the school, and a joint meeting was held with her and the head. These three-cornered conferences, as they came to be called, had several advantages. They enabled the parent to see the school's problem in dealing with the child, and the head to gain insight into the family situation. The avowed purpose of the conference was to reach an understanding about how the child might be helped. Since both the head and the parent participated in its formulation, the former had an interest in carrying out the recommendations within the school and the latter within the home. In no circumstances was any hint uttered that the parent was to blame. If some action by the parent, such as threats of 'putting away' or desertion, was in part responsible for the child's emotional disturbance, its effects were explained in terms of the child's being over-sensitive or taking things too seriously (which would not be going beyond the truth). It was seldom, moreover, that some handicap in the child or some event in history could not be used to encourage an attitude of tolerance in the parent for the child's more tiresome behaviour. Treating the parent as an equal partner in the therapy not only ensured her full cooperation but also often produced expressions of gratitude for the help given and of relief about not being 'put on the carpet'.

The psychologist or School Welfare Officer who has to cover more than one school will probably be able to work most effectively through three-cornered conferences as described above. They have the additional advantage of providing an informal practical training for the head or class teacher who is interested in this aspect of education. In view of the present lack of trained personnel and the size of the problem, it is evident that for the next few years means must be utilized for spreading a general understanding of a therapeutic approach to disturbed behaviour within the school.

Necessity of techniques and special training

Although one comes to admire the skill and human sensitivity of the experienced social worker and of particular heads, it must be realized that these qualities are not sufficient in themselves. The word 'techniques' has been used advisedly to refer to knowledge that depends upon systematic study or training, and for which intuition is no substitute. In the present context it involves the accurate diagnosis of maladjustment and of specific unconscious compulsions such as underlie avoidance behaviour; the recognition of insecurity-producing types of family situation (without which the diagnostician will often miss the basic cause of insecurity completely); and systematic case history-taking that will reveal concomitant neural-somatic impairment. To all this must of course be added a training in therapeutic approaches, of which the not-blaming principle is but one example. In sum, the social worker needs a knowledge of theory and techniques as explicit as those required for the practice of medicine. A service of School Social Workers without specific training of this kind would be of very considerable value but would not yield optimal results. It would be of further advantage if the workers were grouped regionally and had access, preferably through case conferences, to senior caseworkers or psychological consultants. It has also to be recognized that such training is not in general included in the curricula of degree and diploma courses in psychology and social science. It should properly be given in short specialized courses following the general degree or diploma.

As an interim measure, short courses in the handling of maladjusted children and in parent guidance could well be given to selected teachers, who would subsequently be allocated time to enable them to carry out this kind of work. The teacher who undertook the treatment of the exceptionally difficult 'Doris' previously described by the writer[56] was able to exercise effective guidance until the end of the girl's school career and indeed until her marriage. Doris has settled down to become a good wife and mother.

Discipline and the role of the school

It is claimed by some headmasters that troublesome behaviour within the school can be handled, barring the odd case, by good discipline without recourse to psychological or casework methods of treatment. There can be no doubt that what is called the 'general tone' of a school will have a large influence upon the incidence of delinquency and of other deviant behaviour; but the casework and disciplinary approaches must not be regarded as alternatives, nor good discipline equated with reliance upon punishment. From his observation of the striking differences in the amount of delinquency in schools drawing pupils from similar neighbourhoods, A. B. Clegg, Chief Education Officer for the West Riding of Yorkshire, has come to the conclusion that certain heads do possess a mystique of disciplinary ability of which little is known and which the owners do not disclose. He pertinently calls for 'some careful, genuine, sociological investigation of those schools which have really mastered the problem and those which haven't'.[11] He instances a 'blackboard jungle' type of school in which, despite heavy use of corporal punishment, every sort of delinquency and other kinds of deviant behaviour were rife. After five years with a new head the school, which formerly had the highest delinquency rate in the county, had very nearly the lowest – and this was achieved with little caning. The same writer carried out a systematic study[10] of the relationship between caning and delinquency within the schools of his local education authority. A summary of his findings is presented in *Table 7*; the schools are classified in three groups according to their use of corporal punishment. The

Table 7 Corporal punishment related to delinquency rate

Use of corporal punishment within school	*Assessment of general behaviour within school by Div. Educ. Officer*	*Delinquency rate (percentage of pupils appearing in court over previous three years)*
None 9 schools	7 good 2 poor	2·34
Some (up to 2 per cent) 11 schools	7 good 4 poor	2·76
Heavy (over 2 per cent) 10 schools	1 good 9 poor	3·61

Source: Clegg (1961)[10]

heavier the caning, the higher the delinquency rate and the worse the behaviour!

It could have been that certain schools were forced to resort to heavy corporal punishment because they drew their children from underprivileged and somewhat unruly neighbourhoods. With this possible explanation in mind Clegg took as criteria of kind of neighbourhood the rateable value per head of population and the proportion of families living in overcrowded houses. These revealed little difference in the social background of the three groups of schools; indeed, the rateable value per head was least in the schools not using corporal punishment and having the lowest delinquency rate. Clegg does not draw the conclusion that delinquency in the school is directly caused by caning, but that 'attitudes of which excessive caning are symptomatic may be those which induce rebelliousness or which do least to allay or inhibit the tendency towards delinquency which may have its roots in home conditions or elsewhere'.

Summarizing the measures that can be taken within the school to keep delinquency down to a minimum, Clegg enunciates as the first principle that the discipline of the school should be 'the result of carefully thought out principles meticulously worked out in practice'. The examples he gives amount to circumventing as many as possible of the situations conducive to bad behaviour and efficient enforcement of a code of conduct (which included bringing the parents to the school for consultation and guidance). The effect of such a policy is to reduce the amount of stress and the number of temptations and provocations to which the unstable child is exposed. He will be subjected to less bullying and molestation, be less often 'dared' or challenged to participate in foolish or delinquent acts, under less compulsion to misbehave or act the clown in order to win group approbation. It has been seen from the case studies to what extent the inconsequential type of child, who is so common in an underprivileged environment as to pass for a variant of normality, is situation-dominated. The great majority of such children have no intrinsic motivation towards misbehaviour, but are 'easily led'.

Clegg's second principle is that the head should show 'a genuine concern for his pupils as individuals, and a deep compassion directed as much to the Cs and Ds as to the As and Bs'. Children who have developed a readiness for hostility owing to insecurity at home are naturally sensitive to rejection or to being among the non-preferred at school, and will easily slip into an attitude of unconcern for adult approval and adult moral standards. The realization that a hostile child is maladjusted rather than just 'bloody-minded' or a 'bad egg' induces the teacher, sometimes unconsciously, to react with more compassion. The writer has known instances where the teacher's completing a Bristol Guide in respect of a boy has rendered the latter noticeably more amenable and less hostile, although he was of course unaware that any assessment of his behaviour was being made. It was just that the teacher, in the course of completing the form, had come to realize that what he had previously treated as mere bad behaviour was more properly regarded as maladjustment, for which the child could not be held completely responsible.

In brief, Clegg's formula of good discipline combined with compassion will tend to produce conditions under which the vulnerable child has a reasonable chance of adapting himself and of keeping out of trouble. When these conditions do not exist, and hooliganism and delinquency become rife, this is not a matter of the main body of the well-adjusted pupils 'kicking over the traces'. A study of Glasgow boys convicted of vandalism – breaking windows and the glass of bus shelters, damaging trees, etc. – showed that as a group they were somewhat more maladjusted than boys put on probation mainly for theft. In addition to the average of 11 to 14 per cent of boys rated as maladjusted there is a further 16 to 23 per cent in the 'unsettled' class who, under conditions of stress, temptation, and impunity, may indulge in deviant behaviour. The maintenance of high standards of discipline is thus not an alternative remedy to that of individual casework but rather complementary to it and part of the situational treatment of the disturbed child.

Most delinquents are disturbed children

To justify good discipline we do not need to nurse the illusion that all but an insignificant minority of children are 'psychologically normal'. When Mays[40] asserts that 'the vast majority of boys who are brought before the juvenile courts are fundamentally normal personalities', he does so without any factual basis, since he carried out no psychological assessment of the Liverpool club boys who were the subject of his study. His claim that 'perhaps as much as 90 per cent of the total' of offences by juveniles are committed by those of stable personality is contradicted by the findings of systematic studies. A survey of all Glasgow boys put on probation for the first time in 1957 – 78 per cent of them first offenders – showed that, by the standard criterion of 20 or more indications of behaviour disturbance, no less than 46 per cent of them were maladjusted and a further 31 per cent were 'unsettled' or moderately disturbed.[61] Mays's criticism of this finding,[41] to the effect that those put on probation constituted a special group, was invalidated by subsequent results from a 'straight run' of all offenders taken in 1959. This showed that there was no significant difference as regards degree of behaviour disturbance between those boys put on probation (mean maladjustment score 16·9) and those fined (18·0) or admonished (15·9).

It is a mistake, in short, to think that badly behaved boys can be divided into a large majority who are stable and a small minority who are unstable. The distribution of emotional stability is a continuum; consequently the amount of disturbed or 'bad' behaviour that occurs depends upon the amount of stress and instigation provided by the environment. The general assumption of stability and rationality that the law makes is no more true of the 'boy in the street' than it is of the man in the street. The average citizen, if such a term has any meaning, falls a little short of stability, and needs a secure cultural framework to keep him on the path of good behaviour.

A Programme of Practical Measures

A number of measures for dealing with the problems of behaviour disturbance and delinquency can be proposed as a result of experience gained in the course of this study. The first, and central one, upon which the efficient operation of all the others depends, is the establishment of a school-based service of trained Welfare Officers. Nevertheless, such a service does not provide the total answer: the existing Glasgow service was unable to apply the means of treatment indicated for some cases because these were lacking. Adequate discussion of what additional facilities were indicated would take up a book in itself and would involve a survey of numerous pioneer social enterprises, which usually go unreported and receive little publicity. All the present writer can presume to undertake is to list the needs and to mention such few promising experiments as have come to his notice. In order to emphasize that these proposals are given only in outline they are numbered.

1. *A School Welfare Service* is the first need.

2. *Facilities for diagnosis.* When a child is referred to a social agency or is brought before a court for any but a technical offence there should be a systematic diagnostic investigation. This should take into account the likelihood of somatic-neural impairment, and hence of a neural basis for the disturbed behaviour. The neurological examination should not be confined to the testing of the usual reflexes; failure of these may be found in a small number of children who

have suffered gross neural damage, but it would seem that even a minimal impairment or maturational retardation can upset the complicated mechanisms responsible for the control of behaviour. More reliance should consequently be placed upon poor motor co-ordination; thick or jumbled speech; what are popularly called nervous mannerisms; somatic dysfunctions possibly related to failure of homeostasis or of the fine mechanisms responsible for disease resistance; and, finally, evidence of impairment, delayed maturation, or behaviour disturbance in early childhood.

For the delinquent child the application of these diagnostic procedures necessitates a period of remand following the finding of guilt. Remand need not necessarily be to a residential centre in all cases. There is nothing to be said for the present judicial practice in Glasgow, by which young people are brought to court and, if found guilty, sentenced within a few days of the commission of the offence, with only a perfunctory pre-trial investigation. The haphazard results of this system are illustrated in the failure of magistrates to discriminate as to which children will be best dealt with by fining, by probation, or by admonishment; and in their inability to detect future recidivists.[73]

3. *Tutorial provision.* There are certain maladjusted children who cannot be treated within the ordinary school. Although they may be momentarily subdued, punishment is ineffective with them. Upon the inconsequential it makes no lasting impression, and it confirms the hostile in their hostility. The most difficult group of all are those neurally impaired children who react by uncontrolled violence to correction or to everyday frustrations in their dealings with their age-mates. In the present group there was Kenneth, who was removed to an epileptic colony. It is hard to know what solution would have been found if he had not provided the authorities with this opportunity for intervention. (In his whole life he had had only one major and some ten minor fits.) There are other unmanageable children whose impairment remains undiagnosed because it does not show itself in epilepsy. Often their educational backwardness is made the reason for sending them to special schools for the educationally subnormal, where a single such child in a class can make regular teaching difficult.

The London County Council was one of the few authorities in Britain to recognize and make provision for these maladjusted children. In 1945 it established small tutorial classes for them. most of which consist of about six children. The classes are separate from the children's regular schools, some meeting in the district offices of child care or health centres. The principles upon which they work are well described by Margaret Procter, Senior Educational Psychologist to the LCC as it then was:[48]

> 'Each class provides education in an easy informal setting. The group is small enough for there to be a warm intimate relationship between teacher and pupil and for the teacher to permit conduct which would be neither possible nor desirable in the classroom. . . . The child feels secure because of the teacher's tolerant encouraging attitude and because he is accepted by the group no matter what he does. . . . As children are able to accept more discipline, demands made on them are increased until they are ready to accept fully the challenge of an ordinary school.
>
> The child's responsiveness to teaching in a tutorial class varies according to the nature and severity of his handicap. Some children learn quickly in a small group and their progress is accompanied by improved social adaptation. More severely disturbed children cannot learn systematically and at first, learning is incidental. . . .
>
> Since the child is out of his normal school for part of the week, the tutorial class teacher must know exactly what he is missing there. The work of the class must be integrated with the work of the school if each child is to be able to respond fully to his ordinary school when he returns there.'

The tutorial class teacher has the equivalent of one day a week for visits to the parents and for consultation with the children's regular teachers. For these special cases, therefore, the tutorial teacher is able to fulfil the same function as the Glasgow School Welfare Service.

From the above it is evident that a positive policy has been worked out. It is not only that the extremely maladjusted child is likely to be a serious hindrance to the work of an ordinary class; it is recognized that he has educational needs of his own, and as an emotionally handicapped person has a right to treatment even though this may be expensive. The LCC steadily increased the number of its tutorial classes, so that now, as the Inner London Education Authority, it provides this form of treatment for 474 children, most of whom return in due course to their ordinary schools better equipped emotionally and educationally. A city with a population of one million would, to make a similar provision, require some 200 places.

Since the children attend the tutorial classes for half-days, they could be staffed by part-time married women teachers. They would naturally require fairly thorough special training of about a year's duration, such as is provided at present in only a few centres in Britain.

4. *Residential schooling.* For those children who are unlikely to respond even to tutorial provision and family therapy, special residential schools should be maintained as a regular part of the special-schools system, and should indeed have as high a priority as residential schools for the subnormal. They would be required in the first place for those children who are the victims of unconscious compulsions resulting in irrational and sometimes near-psychotic behaviour. Of these by far the commonest – and least recognized – is avoidance-excitement, which is one of the principal motivations of persistent delinquency. The compulsion usually overlies acceptable social attitudes, so that the hectic delinquency is often seen merely as a desire for adventure or a lack of discipline. The first prerequisite of treatment of the acute case is removal from the surroundings that contain reminders of the traumatic experiences. There were two such in the present series, both of whom found their way to approved schools. A third boy, who showed the compulsion to a milder degree, was removed to the care of the local authority because of the threatened violence of the imprisoned father. Another case, in which avoidance-excitement was combined with hostility (the Maltese boy), was cleared up by family therapy.

The second, and larger, category needing residential treatment are the temperamentally vulnerable children in stressful family situations which prove unamenable to the efforts of the caseworkers. In some instances this is a matter of parents who are unable or unwilling to renounce a manner of life that produces acute and chronic insecurity for the child. They include cases of temporary cohabitation, threatened break-up of the family from parental quarrelling, and parental demoralization or social deviance. There were seven in the present sample. In the conferences, family casework was seen to be hopeless, and all that could be done, for lack of any means of voluntary removal of the children concerned, was helplessly to await their progress in delinquency, which would secure their removal. This – in the form of committal to an approved school, placement in the care of the local authority, or a condition of residence in a probation order – duly occurred in six instances. There was evidence that nearly all of these children either consciously wanted removal or unconsciously welcomed it as a means of severing themselves from emotional relationships that had become intolerable. They showed the removal urge and/or the self-banishing hostility that were found in an earlier study[55] to be two of the chief motivations behind persistent delinquency. There was in particular one boy who, by his persistent tiresomeness, destructiveness, and wandering in early childhood and his subsequent home-pilfering, truancy, and running away had become the black sheep of the family. Although his parents were respectable, well-meaning people, he had produced such set attitudes of rejection against himself as could not be mended. He also wanted removal, going in for housebreaking in the mood that he did not care if he were put away; he succeeded in getting to an approved school after, no doubt, causing much inconvenience and nervous shock to his victims and financial loss to their insurance companies.

It is for this group of children, whose maladjustment and delinquency are a result of their own instability combined with unfavourable home conditions, that a new type of residential school is principally needed. The provision of such – together with efficient early detection through a School Welfare Service – could alone significantly reduce the volume of delinquency by removing one of its immediate causes.

The sort of residential school envisaged would need the staff complement of an approved school, as well as a full-time Welfare Officer for home visiting and the services of a psychological adviser. Admission to the school should be subject to the consent of the child and his parents. In most cases consent would easily be obtained from the child, since – as has been seen – removal from the stressful family situation is often the driving force behind hostility and delinquency. Such children are naturally also a trial to their parents, and hence they too would generally not be averse to the idea of residential schooling. Parental consent may not always be forthcoming immediately, but situations are apt to arise when they not only are willing but demand that the child be taken out of the home. As a last resort, it should be possible to make parents see that voluntary entry is preferable, both for their own reputation and for the child's future, to the alternative of allowing the bad behaviour to culminate in committal through the court. From having visited the parents of many boys in approved schools the writer can testify how grateful the majority of them are once the shock of the committal has been overcome. One would expect them to be all the more grateful if the residential schooling or industrial training were offered without the disgrace of committal through the court. In some cases parental consent might have to be obtained to a trial period in the first instance.

When the writer put this proposal for 'voluntary approved schools' to a professional gathering the question was asked: 'But what would we do with the children once we got them there?' The first answer is that the mere 'getting them there' solves many problems – by forestalling the delinquency to which most of the children in question would resort in order to get removed from home; by providing a stable environment that will not be beyond the tolerance of the stress-vulnerable child; by removing inconsequential and affectionally impaired children from temptation and provocation. The minimum requirement is thus an atmosphere of good but not punitive discipline. One might call it a therapeutic discipline based on the principles of minimal stress and the development of normal social attachments. The latter is a prerequisite for the emergence of social obligation and responsibility.

The fostering of social attachments is best done in small family-like units such as in the branches of the National Children's Home. This system consists in making up groups of some eight or nine children, each with its housemother and its own parlour. It means the abandonment of large-scale communal feeding or, if this cannot be avoided, the provision of separate tables for the family groups. It also means the abandonment of large dormitories, three or four children sleeping in one room being the ideal. Mr R. H. Adams, former Principal of the Kingswood classifying school, once remarked to the writer that the only junior approved school to which he could send maladjusted children with the confidence that they would not 'bounce back' was the Coomb School in South Wales, run by the National Children's Home on the above lines. A short time later – as a result of a phase of premature optimism owing to the temporary lessening of delinquency during the early 1950s – the Home Office decided that it would have to be closed, choosing this school because it cost a few more shillings per child per week to run in comparison with other schools, and was a little more expensive in the conveyance of children. That it offered a successful solution to a difficult problem was not taken into account. In an approved school or borstal, where one housemaster has charge of between twenty and forty boys, the development of social attachments is necessarily haphazard. Those who have been rejected have come to expect rejection from other adults and tend to put on a front of hostility or unconcern. Naturally, association with them is unrewarding from the point of view of the adult staff. Similarly, the affectionally impaired boy in whom the need for social attachment awakens during adolescence may not know how to compete for acceptance and affection among a crowd; he is thus likely to remain an isolate, and may rationalize his failure by choosing a life of social deviance. Within a large group, in short, those who most need the opportunity to develop social attachments are denied it. Only when the one-time hostile or affectionless child has learnt to value the affection and approval of the guardian adult will he begin to feel loyalties and moral obligations, and *want* to behave himself. A therapy based upon the building of human attachments and an education in what this implies for the control of behaviour consequently provide a large part of the answer to the query, 'What shall we do with them?' It should be mentioned that there exist residential schools for maladjusted children which work on these principles, but there are too few of them, and they are not generally seen as a form of treatment for delinquent children.

The second major objective of the 'voluntary approved school' should be the reconciliation of the child with his parents in so far as this is possible and advisable. Most instances of violent parental rejection spring from a state of irritable-depressive non-tolerance. This is a form of stress behaviour which, while it lasts, replaces the natural affections, and may even involve physical attack upon the child. In other words, the parent's nerves have gone (to use the popular expression), probably in part as a result of the child's tiresomeness. Once, however, the child is removed from the physical proximity of the overstressed parent, the latter's affections have a chance to revive. It is all too easy, nevertheless, when the parent has other children or the child is a product of an earlier marriage and has jeopardized the present one, for him to be forgotten or 'written off'. A careful treatment plan of reconciliation is therefore needed. In working with a group of housemasters at the Kingswood approved school the writer was able to observe how reacceptance of the boy by the parents could be affected in what seemed at first the most obstinate cases of rejection. For the first year no noticeable progress might be observed, but by the end of the second year reconciliation had been successful. It was agreed that two complete years are usually required: the recent tendency to reduce the length of stay in the approved school militates against success. It also follows that for persistent delinquents – a large proportion of whom have brought upon themselves a degree of parental rejection – committal to a short period of detention is irrelevant to their real needs and a waste of public money.

The practical difficulty of providing and staffing these voluntary schools has to be faced. The courageous thing to do would be to make an experimental conversion of a small number of existing approved schools. This approach would not be so unfeasible, even in view of the present pressure for places at approved schools, since a large proportion of the children attending the experimental schools would be committed to approved schools before long in any case.

5. *Residential industrial training*. The principle of consent can also be applied to the provision of residential industrial training establishments for boys over school age. It is often observed that the youth seeking removal from what to him has become an intolerable home situation first explores sensible means of getting away. Only when, for medical reasons or because of a previous conviction or two, he finds his entry to the army, navy, or merchant navy barred does he make an irrational bid for removal by delinquency.

Those who doubt that such establishments can be successful should visit Turner's Court at Benson in Oxfordshire, of which Colonel R. P. Menday is the present warden. Of the 120 youths in training there, between 40 and 50 per cent have had a history of court appearances, and 60 per cent come under fit person orders from the local authorities. They are thus by no means a selected group of stable youths. The first thing that strikes the visitor is the absence of institutional atmosphere. The domestic quarters are decorated in a cheerful and tasteful contemporary style. Appropriate furniture is provided for each boy's clothing and belongings; there are bright covers on the beds, and reading lamps beside them. The usual size of bedroom holds three, thus avoiding the terrors of a large dormitory. Industrial training groups are of not more than seven or eight under each instructor. The trades taught are agriculture (by very modern methods), building (which provides a good variety of skilled and semi-skilled work), carpentry and wood-machining, painting and decorating, machinery maintenance, and cobbling. The better trainees take up apprenticeships and attend a local technical college for one day a week. Thus, besides its therapeutic function, Turner's Court is also training workers for industries that are short of labour. A measure of its human success is that, at the time of the writer's visit, no one had absconded over the last four years.

The rapid development of provision of this kind is retarded only by a financial anomaly. Half the cost of maintaining a boy in an approved school is paid out of central government funds, but a local authority sending a pre-delinquent boy for residential training of the above type has to meet the whole cost itself. Since at least half the boys committed to approved schools commit their offences in order, at least in part, to secure their removal from home, this amounts to the unwitting encouragement of crime by government subsidy. This last statement is not just an epigrammatic half-truth: it is an application of the more general proposition that a society that provides regular residential treatment for recidivist delinquents but virtually none for pre-delinquents suffers from approximately twice the amount of juvenile crime that need occur.

6. *Leisure-time provision.* The vulnerable, delinquency-prone child should be protected against stress and temptation during his leisure time. This is not only a matter of 'keeping him off the streets' – to use the well-worn phrase – although that is in fact a very important aspect. A free evening with nowhere to go and no money to spend is a nightmare to a semi-literate youth. If his family situation is such as to make an evening at home intolerable he can easily allow himself to fall in with the delinquent frequenters of an amusement arcade or billiard saloon. In the present series it was probably the chronic quarrelling of his parents that finally drove Albert to housebreaking. Geoffrey took to gambling, with what that means in terms of ready money, only when he became unemployed.

For the unsettled or backward boy the highly organized club that aims to maintain good standards is of little use. Either he senses in advance that he would not fit in, or he gets expelled. Clubs that make attendance at an evening class or other organized activity a condition of membership are even less appropriate. The prerequisites are physical warmth, a quiet orderly atmosphere, voluntary recreation, the undemanding companionship of age-peers and of one or more accepted adults. The James Wykeham Youth Club in Bristol has been run successfully along these lines for several years by a group of teachers and social workers, with voluntary classes in reading and handwork. It requires a fairly high ratio of adult helpers to club members, but the attachment to the adult that young people of this type require cannot be provided otherwise. The boys and girls are introduced to the club during their last term or so at school, meet their own teachers there and remain in contact with them over the first years of their employment. If, after a period of habituation to club life, they are considered mature enough, they are introduced to a regular youth club. Such small clubs, at which teachers or social workers can exercise an informal guidance during the difficult post-school years, would form a valuable adjunct to a School Welfare Service.

Providing for the weekend's leisure is more difficult, but just as important, for the delinquency-prone boy. The pioneer weekend residential 'club' at Northorpe Hall near Leeds is worth watching as a possible prototype, not only as a solution to the stresses and temptations of the weekend period, but also as a means of providing opportunities for re-education. Probation officers in Leeds and the staff of Northorpe Hall chose thirty-six boys, in the first place, for a three-week holiday in Malvern; subsequently the boys have spent monthly weekends in rotation (from Friday night to Monday morning) at the Hall. In addition, many of them spend a part of their summer holidays there, and most of those over fourteen come for midweek classes in the Duke of Edinburgh's Award Scheme and stay the night. Thus the Hall provides a kind of residential club which brings its members under the influence of socially-minded adults and gives them the opportunity of a relief from the stresses of unsatisfactory homes.

At the time of selection all the boys were on probation, and none was excluded because of difficult behaviour or because of inconvenient habits such as bedwetting. Their ages on selection ranged from ten to fourteen, with an average of eleven and a half, so that they were approaching the age of greatest delinquency proneness. Nevertheless, their offences during the fifteen months of their attachment to the scheme have been below expectation for boys put on probation. None has persisted in delinquency to a degree that resulted in committal to an approved school (of the three who did in fact go to approved schools, two committed their offences prior to entry to the scheme and one was beyond the control of his mother).

There was no evidence of 'delinquent infection' or of using acquaintance with other delinquents for the planning of gang exploits. Those who have had experience of young offenders in a free environment can testify that the spreading or planning of delinquency in this way occurs only when the young people are in an antisocial, hostile mood; it is signally absent during periods when they appreciate the availability of a friendly adult. One likely reason for the absence of persistent delinquency among the chosen boys was that they had no need to commit offences in order to secure removal from an intolerable emotional situation. Northorpe Hall was always at hand, and they have often telephoned for advice or just to gain strength from the contact. Two boys made their way thither by a seven-hour foot-slog when pressure was put on them to join in an exploit of a delinquent gang, and one boy – after a series of unsuccessful placements with foster mothers – made his home there. The conveyance of boys to and from their homes in a minibus gives opportunities to the warden and his helpers to get to know the parents and to carry out informal family therapy. It has to be an exceedingly hard-hearted or indifferent parent not to respond to someone who is doing something for his or her child, and a weekend residential centre might make openings where routine casework visits fail.

Owing to financial limitations Northorpe Hall has to be run on somewhat substandard lines, with voluntary student weekend helpers, and the verdict of many official visitors is that it is one of those special arrangements that depend upon the inspiration and dedication of individuals. Nevertheless, we should seriously consider the idea of residential clubs, where children could find refuge from the stresses and temptations of city life.

7. *The school's contribution.* The part that the school can play has already been discussed earlier in this chapter. Suffice it to note here that if the teacher is to be able to provide guidance during the last years at school and in some cases in the post-school years he must renounce diciplinary procedures which place a barrier between him and the growing boy or girl. Corporal punishment is in any case usually ineffective with the disturbed child, and ethically indefensible with those – perhaps the majority – whose disturbance is fundamentally a matter of neural impairment.

8. *Application of research findings.* The last proposal is of a general character: it is that, instead of the periodic wringing of hands that passes for concern about juvenile deviance, the facts of the problem as revealed by recent research be taken account of and acted upon. It is true that because so much research has had to be conducted with inadequate resources it has not been as systematic or on as large a scale as its authors would have liked. But it is no longer true that we are ignorant of the causes of juvenile delinquency. Research workers will always dispute over unsettled issues at the boundaries of knowledge, and each new major finding poses new queries. Nevertheless, if a delinquency-prevention programme framed upon what we do

know were put into operation the volume of juvenile crime could be reduced to a small fraction of what it is now. The justification for this apparently rash claim is that the most cursory appraisal of current measures shows to what extent the wrong things are being done. Measures that are naïvely assumed to deter in fact encourage the commission of offences. Money is spent at too late a stage, when the boy or youth has already chosen, or been forced on to, a path of crime. In ethical and human terms, as well as in those of pure economics, we are spending public money badly.

How can we counter this, knowing that the waste is not just due to inertia or incompetence, but to a fear of deep-lying public misunderstandings and prejudices about the nature of crime? The idea that the troublesome child is likely to be emotionally handicapped in the same literal sense that another child can be spastic or mentally handicapped will not be easily accepted. It is, in short, a question of whether any governing group will have the courage to carry the theme of the scientific age into this thorny field.

Part of the answer will undoubtedly be to establish the facts by a series of impeccably designed researches supported by adequate personnel and finance. But for the findings we should have to wait perhaps five years, and meantime the problem grows. Such studies must nevertheless be undertaken, because they will add to the precision of our knowledge as well as render the main principles incontrovertible.

What is needed now, however, is practical demonstration of the effectiveness of the measures indicated by current research. The writer would like to suggest that the proposals outlined above be initiated, as a piece of operational research, in a single city. As they were established their effects upon the delinquency rate could be observed. If it were found that the cost of the measures were comparable with the money saved from less damage to property, fewer young people in approved schools and borstals, fewer young adults in prison, and – last but not least – fewer social misfits and unemployables, the programme could be applied on a national scale.

PART II

Truants

CHAPTER SEVEN

A Study of Truants

In 1961 the Education Welfare Officers' National Association asked the writer to undertake with them a research into truancy. A pilot study was initiated in Sheffield and Salford, but although its results were encouraging no further progress could be made owing to lack of finance. Some two years later, however, the writer was invited by the United Nations Educational, Scientific, and Cultural Organization to conduct a validation of his Delinquency Prediction Instrument. This project required a sample of boys and girls selected from all over Britain, among whom would be a goodly proportion of the delinquency prone. A sample of truants with controls of the same age would meet this requirement admirably. It was consequently agreed that the two research projects should be amalgamated. The marriage was a particularly happy one, since the Education Welfare Officers were in contact with both the schools and the homes, and it is part of their duties to know the whereabouts of children and to send notification when a child moves from one local administrative area to another. In addition, their Association agreed to undertake the whole of the detailed administration of the research, and this they did with admirable efficiency.

Design of the Research

Those Education Welfare Officers who agreed to take part were asked to select their two most recent truants, as far as possible choosing one from the primary stage of education (between 5 and 11–12 years of age) and one from the secondary stage (between 11–12 and 15 years). Since some of the officers had difficulty in finding two recent truants a few selected a third or a fourth; the net result was that the

305 truants who were the subject of study were supplied by 168 Welfare Officers scattered throughout Britain.

Two controls were selected for each truant from within the same school. The first was the child of the same sex born on the same day as the truant, or the day nearest to it. If two or more children were equally near the birth-date the one whose name was earliest in the alphabet was chosen. These, named the birth-date controls, formed a reasonably representative sample of British schoolchildren.

Cultural or individual deviance

The second control was chosen in order to obtain a measure of cultural influences. It has been fashionable in recent years to characterize much social deviance not as individual waywardness but as the ordinary behaviour of boys and girls within certain subcultures: the typical delinquent is regarded as a well-adjusted boy who is merely conforming to the delinquent and crime-tolerant atmosphere of his inner-urban neighbourhood. It is not denied that such an atmosphere does exist *among certain groups* in certain urban localities and that in some cities there are 'black spots' where families containing delinquents congregate. But we are not justified in concluding that the prevalence of crime in these districts is merely a matter of local tradition.

That cultural factors are ultimately determinative is shown by the growth of delinquency in modern industrial centres and its rarity in non- or pre-industrial cultures. But the reasons go deeper than the mere creation of a crime-tolerant atmosphere. The incidence of congenital, including neural, defect is much higher among underprivileged social groups; and cultural disintegration brings with it a great deal of family insecurity. For these two reasons we would expect to find much more behaviour disturbance among juveniles living in underprivileged areas.*

Not all delinquents (in the sense of young people who have been found guilty of what for adults would be called crimes) are disturbed, and not all disturbed young people are delinquents. But delinquents have been found to be between four and five times more prone to maladjustment than other boys in the same schools.[61] Those, like Mays, who have tried to explain social deviance mainly in terms of the direct transmission of delinquent attitudes, have tried to discount this finding by arguing that the behaviour rated as maladjusted upon

* For a fuller statement of the cultural determinants of delinquency and maladjustment, see Stott.[68, 73]

the Bristol Social Adjustment Guides (the instrument used in the study of delinquents referred to above) was merely the typical behaviour of boys living in neighbourhoods where people's ideas about right and wrong are quite different from those embodied in the BSAG. If this is true of one sort of social deviant we should expect it to be true of another; in the type of neighbourhood where stealing is regarded lightly, no great store would be placed upon school attendance. If the typical delinquent within the underprivileged neighbourhood is a well-adjusted boy following the local pattern of life, we should expect this to apply even more to the truant.

This view could be tested by choosing a second control for each truant – a child of the same sex and year-group, who lived in the same street, or as near as could be found. These neighbourhood controls, as they were called, would thus in the main be subjected to the same cultural influences as the truants, and they would all – taking the same route to and from school every day – have known each other personally.

The scores of the three samples on the Bristol Social Adjustment Guides would thus make possible two crucial comparisons. The differences between the neighbourhood controls and the truants should show the extent to which the latter were affected by some individual factor of behaviour disturbance, apart from any tradition of bad behaviour within the neighbourhood. And the differences between the two sets of controls should show what element in the scores was due to a specifically cultural factor characteristic of the neighbourhoods where the truants lived.

Intrinsic Disturbance of Truants

The results, in terms of mean BSAG scores, are shown for boys and girls separately in *Tables 8* and *9*. The Delinquency Prediction scores, abstracted from the BSAG scores, are also given. The BSAG means for the controls are so different from the means for the truants, in the case of both boys and girls, that statistical tests of significance are unnecessary; however, for the record, they are included in the tables.*

* The reader unversed in statistics may appreciate a short explanation of the measure of significance employed. A difference between two means, or averages, may be due to a real difference in the samples, such as would be likely to recur in further samples selected in the same manner from the same population; or

Table 8 Behaviour disturbance among boy truants and controls

	N	*Mean BSAG score*	*Mean Delinquency Prediction score*
All boy truants	220	24·93	29·55
Birth-date controls	214	7·38	3·60
Neighbourhood controls	216	8·53	3·78
		Critical ratio	*p*
Truants/birth-date controls		17·649	$<$·001
Truants/neighbourhood controls		15·996	$<$·001
Birth-date/neighbourhood controls		1·449	n.s.

The BSAG scores are made up of the number of indications of behaviour disturbance marked by the teacher in respect of each child. *Table 8* shows that the mean score for the boy truants is well above 20, which is taken as the borderline of maladjustment, whereas those for both groups of controls fall below 9, which is the upper limit for quasi-stability. We have to conclude, therefore, that there is some individual factor of behavioural instability, amounting to 16·40 points, that distinguishes the truants from other boys in their neighbourhoods, whether or not the latter happened to be truant or otherwise socially deviant. The high scores for the truants, and by

it may be a fortuitous one, arising from the particular samples chosen. If, for example, another 220 boy truants were similarly chosen, it would be very unlikely indeed that their mean BSAG score would come out at exactly 24·93. On the other hand, we should not expect it to be widely different unless there were a specific reason such as, say, a sudden raising in the meantime of the school-leaving age to 18 years. If the mean score for this second group of truants was 22 or 27, we should need some way of estimating whether the difference was due to the chances of sampling or to the intrusion of some other factor. The method employed is the critical ratio, which compares the difference between the means with a measure of the amount of variation in the scores.

The traditional level of statistical significance is reached when the difference of the means is approximately twice the above-mentioned measure of variation, giving a critical ratio of 2. At this level (to be precise, 1·960 for samples of the size used in the present survey) the probability (p) of such a difference occurring by chance is one in twenty (or ·05). The higher the critical ratio the smaller the risk of a chance difference, and the greater the significance. Thus, if the ratio is more than 2·576, p is less than one in a 100 ($<$ ·01); if it is more than 3·291, p is less than one in a 1000 ($<$ ·001). The level of significance given by p $<$ ·001 is the highest that it is considered worth while to record, since it amounts to virtual certainty that the result is not a chance one. In fact, the values of the critical ratios in the present study would make the risk of a chance result less than one in a million.

extension for delinquents, cannot, in short, be discounted as a cultural artifact.

The extent of a possible cultural distortion, if any, in the BSAG scores is seen by the small excess, of 1·15, in the mean for the neighbourhood over the birth-date controls. This difference is below the level of statistical significance, but it probably does reflect a slightly greater prevalence of behaviour disturbance in a somewhat less privileged social environment. It would indeed be surprising if this were not so, considering the higher incidence of most forms of defect among underprivileged social groups.

The mean Delinquency Prediction score for the truants puts them near the boundary of the 52 and 82 per cent chance of delinquency as estimated from the Glasgow probation study.[65] The Prediction scores for the controls give a 14 per cent chance by this criterion. In a total year-group of Glasgow school-leavers Ferguson[16] found that 12·2 per cent had at some time been convicted in a court, so that the above prognosis, with a possible slight bias towards lower social class, is not unfeasible.

Table 9 Behaviour disturbance among girl truants and controls

	N	*Mean BSAG score*	*Mean Delinquency Prediction score*
All girl truants	85	24·14	29·18
Birth-date controls	85	7·53	4·27
Neighbourhood controls	84	6·13	2·54
		Critical ratio	*p*
Truants/birth-date controls		10·878	<·001
Truants/neighbourhood controls		12·429	<·001
Birth-date/neighbourhood controls		1·148	n.s.

Both the BSAG and the Delinquency Prediction scores for the girl truants are surprisingly similar to those of the boys. However, the tendency, seen among the boys, for the neighbourhood to score slightly higher than the birth-date controls does not hold for girls, the position being reversed for them. Once again, the difference is not significant statistically, therefore it would be fruitless to try to account for it. It should, however, be borne in mind that girls suffer less congenital impairment than boys, so that they would be less affected by an underprivileged environment. The results for the boy and girl controls viewed as a whole show a satisfactory homogeneity, which indicates that the Bristol Guides are reasonably free of cultural and sex bias. We may therefore conclude that the behaviour disturbance they measure is in the main of an individual character.

Halo effect?

It has been suggested that the very high scores obtained by delinquents on the BSAG are due to what is called 'teacher prejudice' or a halo effect: knowing that they are delinquent, the teachers tend to mark other bad things about them. This accusation is implausible for several reasons. The marking of the BSAG does not entail any interpretation, or rating on a scale ranging from good to bad or desirable to undesirable. Within each area of behaviour the teacher chooses a descriptive word or phrase describing the objective reaction of the child. Thus the teacher's attention is concentrated upon a number of concrete alternatives, which give little scope for prejudgement. Second, it is often forgotten by psychologists, especially those who have never taught, that the day-to-day work of the teacher involves innumerable acts of discernment about the way in which individual children behave, so that his discriminatory powers become sharpened by practice. One cannot hold discussions with teachers without appreciating this, and it is an unwarranted slur upon a professional group to suggest that they would be actuated by blind prejudice. Nevertheless, it is important to deal with objections of the above type systematically since one's knowlege of a situation remains a personal matter and other people cannot be expected to accept uncritically judgements based thereon. A lucky accident helped to refute the charge of prejudice in the truancy survey. In fourteen instances the teachers revealed that they were not aware that the boys in question were truants, since they did not mark them as such on the Bristol Guide. If the remainder of the truants had obtained high scores because of teacher prejudice, we should expect the scores for these boys to be much lower. In fact, the mean score for them was 21·42. This is 3·5 points lower than for the truants as a whole, but one point should be added to their score for the fact of truancy. The difference is not statistically significant, and the mean for the fourteen truants remains nearly three times higher than the means for the controls. It is therefore improbable that the high scores for the truants as a whole were spurious.

Background to Truancy

The Education Welfare Officers, for their part, completed a schedule for each truant covering the frequency of and reasons for the truancy; the extent to which the truant was also delinquent; parental attitudes to school attendance and education; the condition of the truant's home; and the composition and structure of the family. The Officers were in a good position to provide such information, since – apart from their chief responsibility of ensuring school attendance – they often gain insight into home conditions by acting as unofficial family advisers and caseworkers (this indeed being probably the most valuable part of their job).

Reasons for truanting

This part of the survey yielded some results that ran counter to popular expectation. It has often been assumed that much truancy is due merely to a dislike of the monotony of school by active, adventure-loving boys. One hears also of cases of older boys 'cutting school' in order to view a sporting event on television or perhaps to attend the event in person. *Table 10* shows that there is no evidence that such types of truancy are indulged in by stable and otherwise well-behaved boys and girls. It is of course possible that some are stable and clever enough not to get caught, or that if they are their truancy is dealt with by the headmaster and not reported to the Welfare Officer. Nevertheless, the high mean score for those who were known by the Welfare Officer to have truanted because of some special attraction suggests that there is no 'normal' type of truancy. Although, on the surface, it may seem excusable for a boy to stay at home to view a sporting event, a little thought makes one appreciate that such a boy would tend to have little loyalty to his teachers and to regard them as an outside group. Unless his parents condone his cutting school, it must be assumed that he has little regard for them either.

The third comparison in *Table 10* shows that little credence must be given to a dislike of the school or of a teacher as a reason or justification for truancy. Children who proffer this excuse may in fact feel such dislikes, but these are probably symptomatic of their own unhappiness; stable children do not truant, or indulge in other seriously deviant behaviour, because they dislike some element in the school situation.

Table 10 Reasons for truanting: boys and girls

Reason for truanting	*N*	*BSAG score*	*Delinquency Prediction score*
1. To see a special attraction (sporting event, etc.)	24	25·46	33·33
Because pals wanted him to	27	28·96	31·41
Critical ratio		0·973	0·266
p		n.s.	n.s.
2. To see a special attraction (with no upsetting circumstances)	24	25·54	33·12
Because of some upset at school or at home	68	25·99	30·96
Critical ratio		0·137	0·321
p		n.s.	n.s.
3. To see a special attraction (with no dislike of school)	21	23·76	32·52
Dislike of school	103	26·64	32·60
Critical ratio		0·907	0·011
p		n.s.	n.s.

First-time and recidivist truants

There were smaller differences than expected between those who had truanted only once and the occasional and persistent truants. The first comparison of *Table 11* shows that the first-timers get significantly lower scores than the persistent truants, but their mean is nonetheless above the criterion score for maladjustment. Many of the first-timers would be at the beginning of a bout of truancy, and this probably accounts for the small difference between the occasional and more persistent truants as shown in the second comparison. On the other hand, the Prediction scores rise significantly with the amount of truancy. The persistent truant marks himself out as a child in urgent need of treatment. It is also of interest that those truants who absent themselves for single days (comparison 3) are somewhat more maladjusted and delinquency prone than those who do so for several days together. But this is probably a reflection of the tendency to greater disturbance in those (*Table 10*) who yielded to invitations to truant or who truanted with companions (*Table 12*).

Table 11 Frequency of truanting: boys and girls

Frequency of truanting	*N*	*BSAG score*	*Delinquency Prediction score*
1. Only once	47	21·17	19·85
On and off, or had had earlier phase	209	26·04	31·72
Critical ratio		2·520	4·358
p		approx. ·01	<·001
2. Once or twice	35	23·14	23·31
More than twice	221	25·31	30·74
Critical ratio		1·015	2·127
p		n.s.	<·05
3. For single days	101	27·14	32·16
For several days on end	177	24·13	28·97
Critical ratio		2·023	1·081
p		<·05	n.s.

Solitary and gang truants

The lower scores for the solitary truants, as shown in *Table 12*, were again contrary to expectation; but the differences were of degree within the range of marked maladjustment and delinquency proneness. Possibly the solitary truants included a few children who feared to come to school because they anticipated some punishment or disagreeable encounter with another pupil. The very high mean scores for the gang truants finally dispose of the notion that within certain subcultures seriously deviant behaviour is indulged in by well-adjusted young people. Those who truanted with others would already have found their 'birds of a feather', and this is characteristic also of the hostile, antisocial type of delinquent.

Table 12 Companionship in truanting: boys and girls

Companionship in truanting	*N*	*BSAG score*	*Delinquency Prediction score*
Truanted alone	139	24·95	29·80
Truanted with others	125	30·28	35·86
Critical ratio		5·106	2·312
p		<·001	approx. ·02

Delinquent and non-delinquent truants

The truants who were also socially deviant by way of formal delinquency would be expected to reveal themselves as more disturbed and delinquency prone than the non-delinquent. This is confirmed in *Table 13,* and these results afford a measure of validation for the Delinquency Prediction Instrument. The difference of 9 points between the Prediction means for the two groups compared with only a 3½-point difference in the BSAG means shows that this instrument tends to pick out symptoms that are more characteristic of delinquents, and that it can do this even within a highly deviant group such as truants.

Table 13 Delinquent and non-delinquent truants

Delinquency record	*N*	*BSAG score*	*Delinquency Prediction score*
Found guilty of one or more offences	79	26·99	36·09
No offence known	201	23·49	26·74
Critical ratio		2·143	2·942
p		<·05	<·01

Parental attitudes

The attitudes of parents to school attendance and to their children's education are useful indicators of cultural group. It is seen from *Tables 14* and *15* that a considerable proportion of truants have parents who, while realizing that their children should attend school, do not take a very serious view of their truancy and show little interest in their children's progress. If truancy is just 'the done thing' in this cultural group, we should expect the truants in question to show themselves as reasonably stable young people, or at any rate to have lower scores than those who truant in defiance of parental discipline.

In fact *Table 14* shows the opposite to be the case: the truants with easygoing parents were more maladjusted than those with strongly disapproving parents. Although significant, the differences in the mean scores were not great, so that we are not justified in presuming a causal relationship. The explanation is probably that within the cultural group where little importance is attached to school attendance there would be a greater amount of family stress.

Table 14 Parental attitudes to truancy

Parental attitudes to truancy	*N*	*BSAG score*	*Delinquency Prediction score*
Parents condone or do not take a serious view	150	26·54	32·54
Parents very angry, threaten hidings, etc.	114	22·28	25·35
Critical ratio		2·858	2·680
p		$<$·01	$<$·01

The same could also account for the higher scores of those truants whose parents take no interest in their education (*Table 15*). Such parents tend to follow a happy-go-lucky, hedonistic pattern of life, and think rather in terms of having the maximum number of the family bringing in money than in terms of apprenticeship. Jephcott and Carter[30] have reported that in families with this kind of outlook there is likely to be less marital stability and less security for the children. It is interesting that the lowest mean BSAG score is that for the truants belonging to education-conscious social groups. This result could be due to a cultural factor in the BSAG, but even so the difference in scores is seen to be small: only some 1·5 points differentiate the truants whose parents are concerned about their education from those who are members of typical working-class families, and their score is 5·2 points below the mean of those who belong to the educationally indifferent social strata. The latter result is consistent with the finding that delinquents living in homes of inadequate standard tend to be more maladjusted than those in adequate-standard homes.[68] This evidence runs directly contrary to theories of neighbourhood infection, but it is in accordance with the observation of a greater amount of general maladjustment[61] and of all types of defect in underprivileged social groups.

Table 15 Parental attitudes to education

Parental attitudes to education	*N*	*BSAG score*	*Delinquency Prediction score*
1. Want child to learn, but are not ambitious on his behalf	63	22·61	24·44
Take no interest; unaware of child's progress at school; yet realize he ought to attend	179*	26·34	32·57
Critical ratio		2·119	2·770
p		·05	·01
2. Want child to get on, and show a sensible interest	44	21·11	22·59
Take no interest; unaware of child's progress at school; yet realize he ought to attend	185*	26·32	32·35
Critical ratio		2·682	3·115
p		·01	·01

* The discrepancy between these totals is explained by the fact that a number of cases were excluded in which the Welfare Officer marked both alternatives in the first comparison.

Whatever the explanation of the differences between the mean scores for the three cultural groups represented in *Table 15*, they are not large when compared with those for the controls, and in no group does the mean fall below the score of 20 taken as the criterion for maladjustment. Once again it is seen that the truants belonging to the lower cultural groups tend to be more maladjusted.

Standard of home

The condition of the home is another good indicator of cultural group, and here if anywhere we should have expected to find a cultural factor in the BSAG scores. The differences in the mean scores of truants from high-standard homes and truants from low-standard homes reveal the same trend as the scores for parental attitudes to school attendance and interest in education, but they do not reach significance (*Table 16*). Such as they are, they run counter to the notion that even truancy can be regarded as the well-adjusted behaviour of boys within a subculture that rejects the norms of the dominant culture.

Table 16 Truants' home conditions

Condition of home	*N*	*BSAG score*	*Delinquency Prediction score*
1. Reasonably clean	153	23·95	27·88
Spick and span	25	23·76	26·20
Critical ratio		0·071	0·444
p		n.s.	n.s.
2. Untidy, low standard, poor	89	25·36	32·42
Critical ratio (relating (2) to 'reasonably clean')		0·883	1·410
p		n.s.	n.s.
3. Very dirty or utterly demoralized	33	26·85	31·12
Critical ratio (relating (3) to 'reasonably clean')		1·74	0·658
p		n.s.	n.s.

The general picture is of a surprising sameness in the amount of behaviour disturbance and of delinquency proneness in truants from all classes of home. The most feasible explanation of this is that truancy is a form of behavioural breakdown that occurs when the degree of stress exceeds the tolerance threshold of the individual child. There is then a reversion to a pattern of stress behaviour which varies little as between one cultural group and another.

The kinds of stressful family situation that are conducive to breakdown are by no means found only in underprivileged or culturally disintegrated social groups. They are met more frequently in the former, and much more so in the latter; but the main bulk of delinquents come from ordinary working-class families with adequate domestic standards. Of the Glasgow delinquents placed on probation only 22 per cent could be definitely classified as living in culturally substandard homes, compared with 59 per cent in homes of average or superior standard.[68] If we judge by the material condition of the home, the proportions were not very different for the truants: exactly half of them had reasonably clean homes, to which must be added the 8 per cent in the 'spick and span' class; there were 29 per cent in untidy, low-standard homes, and only 11 per cent in culturally demoralized families.

Familial truanting

Nearly half of the truants had brothers or sisters who had also truanted. If a family situation is rendering one child maladjusted there is a higher probability that siblings will be similarly affected. The tendency for siblings also to be truants is therefore consistent with the view that truancy is a symptom of breakdown under stress. However, it is also consistent with an explanation in terms of cultural suggestion, since brothers and sisters, even more than children in different families, are likely to have the same social attitudes and behavioural norms. But there is no reason to suppose that those, if any, who truant merely as a matter of family tradition will be more or less maladjusted than other children in their neighbourhood. If, consequently, a significant number of such sibling-led truants exist, the mean score of the 'familial' type should be lower than that for other truants. The finding was in the contrary direction (*Table 17*). That the difference does not reach statistical significance suggests once more that truancy occurs at a breakdown point signalled by a fairly large number of symptoms, and is seldom a casual occurrence or just something that children within a family copy from one another.

Table 17 Truants with truanting siblings

Truants	*N*	*BSAG score*	*Delinquency Prediction score*
With brother or sister truant	131	25·85	31·55
With no sibling truant	139	23·61	27·23
Critical ratio		1·51	1·56
p		n.s.	n.s.

Broken homes

In the Glasgow probation survey the delinquents from broken homes were hardly more maladjusted than those living in intact families (BSAG scores of 20·8 and 19·7 respectively).[74] Similarly, among the truants the fact in itself of a broken home seemed to have little effect upon the level of maladjustment. Indeed, from *Table 18* it is seen that those living with both parents had slightly, but not significantly, higher scores than those living with one parent only or with neither parent. It appears that if the family situation is such as to give rise to feelings of anxiety or rejection, and the child has the sort of temperament that is affected thereby, the formal structure of the family is immaterial.

Table 18 Family structure and maladjustment

Truants	*N*	*BSAG score*	*Delinquency Prediction score*
Living with both parents	191	25·35	29·61
Living with mother only	71	23·24	28·69
Living with father only	24	24·21	29·63
Living with own parent and step-parent	13	21·85	25.54
Foster children	6	31·83	45·17
Total not living with both parents	114	23·67	29·22

Summary and Conclusions

Severe maladjustment of truants

The mean score for the truants was nearly three times that for the neighbourhood controls, and over three times that for the birth-date controls. Some 63 per cent of the truants were maladjusted compared with only 10·4 per cent of the controls as a whole. This large difference, illustrated in *Figure 1*, is in striking contrast to the slight or moderate differences between the various groups of truants. The largest intra-truant difference – between those whose parents took a sensible interest in their education and those whose parents were indifferent – amounted to only 25 per cent. Even though the truants who were in addition delinquent were significantly more disturbed, in a statistical sense, than those who were not convicted of an offence, the actual difference in score amounted to only 15 per cent.

No 'normal' type of truancy – just 'cutting school' because of some outside attraction – could be identified, and boys who indulged in truancy on these grounds were on average as maladjusted as those who truanted for other alleged reasons.

The theory that much social deviance is the typical behaviour of well-adjusted young people in certain neighbourhoods was seen to be without foundation. The controls who lived in the same neighbourhoods as the truants were little if any more disturbed than controls selected randomly from the same schools.

Figure 1 SOCIAL ADJUSTMENT OF TRUANTS AND CONTROLS

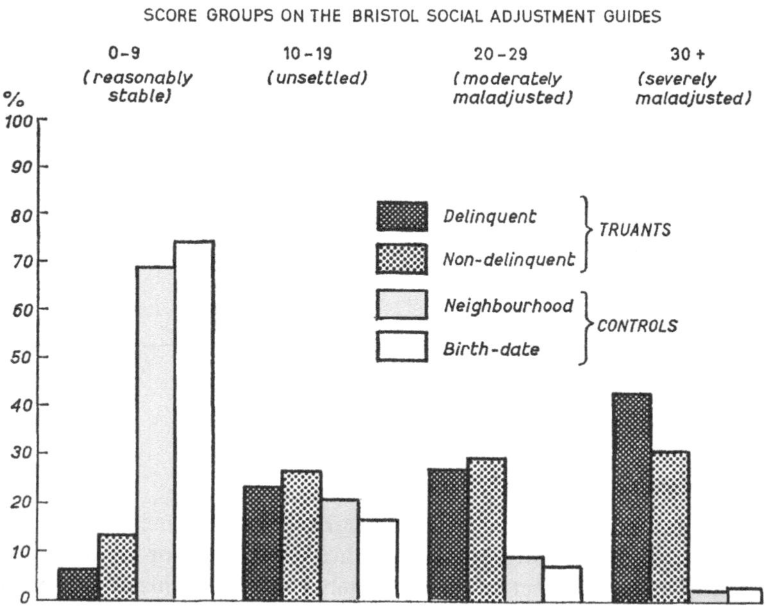

The truants who belonged to underprivileged or education-undervaluing families were slightly more disturbed, although the theory of cultural infection as put forward by Mays would have predicted the reverse. On the other hand, all the evidence supports the view that truancy is in the main a symptom of a fairly general behaviour disturbance. Those truants belonging to families or social groups in which the likelihood of insecurity or other stress was greater tended to be more maladjusted. Nevertheless, the relative constancy of the level of behaviour disturbance for all types of truant suggested that truancy was characteristic of a certain stage of breakdown. This stage seems to be consistent with the concept of a reversion to a pattern of stress behaviour once the tolerance threshold of the individual has been overstepped.

Truants an impaired and vulnerable group

In the following chapter evidence is quoted to show that this tolerance threshold is significantly lower when signs of other impairment are present. Proneness to ill health or physical defect brings with it a greater chance of temperamental instability, and hence of vulnerability to stress. It will be seen that this correlation is most marked in normal groups such as the controls of the truants. Among them there will be a minority of vulnerable individuals who have been subjected to stress up to the point where they show one of the typical patterns of stress behaviour. Since, however, truancy is so characteristic of a high degree of maladjustment, it may well be that the great majority of truants are temperamentally impaired individuals. If this is so, there would be no great difference in degree of maladjustment between those truants who happened to show some additional evidence of impairment and those whose impairment took only a behavioural form. It will be seen later (*Table 27*, p. 136 below) that, in the truants as a group, the unhealthy were only slightly more maladjusted than the healthy. But, compared with the controls, 70 per cent more truants suffered from respiratory complaints and 140 per cent more from other forms of ill health.

Even though common impairments tend to be found in association, it does not follow that a child suffering from one type necessarily suffers from others. If a child is temperamentally impaired there may be, say, a 30 per cent risk of a health handicap. If only a proportion of the truants were impaired and the rest were what might be described as neuro-physically intact, we should expect to find the usual tendency for the more disturbed to have more ill health. *Table 19* shows this not to be the case. In contrast to the controls, there is little difference in the numbers of unhealthy truants in each of the BSAG score categories.

Table 19 Behaviour disturbance and ill health

	BSAG score category		
	Stable and quasi-stable (0–9)	*Unsettled (10–19)*	*Maladjusted (20+)*
ALL TRUANTS			
Number in BSAG category	35	76	194
Percentage with respiratory complaint	31·4	19·7	27·3
Percentage with other ailment	17·1	19·7	22·2
ALL CONTROLS			
Number in BSAG category	283	144	172
Percentage with respiratory complaint	4·3	15·9	22·2
Percentage with other ailment	2·5	13·0	18·1

The fact that among the truants the health impairments are not associated with more severe behaviour disturbance must mean that the BSAG scores do not serve to pick out those who have suffered multiple impairment. Considering the inexorable nature of the latter tendency and the large amount of ill health among the truants, this could be the case only if nearly all truants belong to the multiple-impaired category. Such an explanation is strengthened by the small number of truants – less than 11·5 per cent – who came in the stable and quasi-stable groups (BSAG scores of 0–9) compared with 71 per cent of the controls. We are not even justified in assuming that this small proportion of low-scoring truants were all in fact reasonably stable. It must be born in mind that the BSAG scores register overt behaviour disturbance such as can be observed by a teacher who knows the child reasonably well. A certain number of emotionally disturbed children, especially those who sit quiet in class and day-dream most of the time, may give few overt signs, and in other cases the teachers may have been new to the class and not have had an opportunity to get to know the children in question. It is probable, therefore, that the above percentage overstates the proportion of reasonably well-adjusted truants.

Social and educational implications

The central feature of truancy has been seen to be one of fairly severe maladjustment among a class of temperamentally vulnerable children exposed to a degree of stress which exceeded their emotional reserves. The traditional remedies of punishment, admonition, fining the parents, and so on are irrelevant. It is no longer a question primarily of getting the unwilling pupil to school or of enforcing attendance within sections of the population that are indifferent to the advantages of education. In some cases these remedies may even be harmful. One of the Education Welfare Officers sent in a personal report about a former truant, in an extremely distressing family situation, who was caned by his headmaster for smoking. This was the signal for a round of breaking into premises and repeated arson, culminating in fire damage of over £100,000 to a factory. In mitigation of the headmaster's disciplinary measure, he probably knew little about the boy's home circumstances or of the patient efforts of the Welfare Officer to help him to overcome them. If there had been a School Welfare Officer as a regular member of the staff, with primary responsibility for the handling of children in difficulty, such an independent action and its unfortunate outcome could have been avoided.

If responsibilities of this kind are to be conferred upon Welfare Officers, they must be formally qualified in family casework, either by initial training or by opportunities for later in-service qualification. The cost of such a service would certainly be much less than the social loss and expense of allowing maladjusted children to form, as they grow up, a shiftless, neurotic, or delinquent section of the community.

PART III

Towards an Understanding of Behaviour Disturbance

CHAPTER EIGHT

A Law of Multiple Congenital Impairment

Multiple Impairment among the Mentally Retarded

The frequency of multiple handicap has long been recognized by those who have administrative responsibilities: the educationally backward child may also be emotionally disturbed, the deaf also partially sighted, the delinquent enuretic. The sheer fact of this tendency to multiple handicap thus needs little formal demonstration.

Ill health in infancy

Among 102 mentally retarded children, selected on account of their normal physical appearance – that is, excluding those who were mongols or patently deformed – 56 (55 per cent) had had at least one serious non-epidemic illness during their first three years of life.[57] Only 18 per cent of the 450 mentally normal controls had been similarly unhealthy in infancy. The diseases in question were for the most part those of the respiratory and digestive systems, failure to gain weight or wasting away, extreme feebleness or an ailing condition in the first months, proneness to local infections, abscesses or skin complaints. The 56 children had between them 85 unhealthy conditions, or 1·5 each; in them the presence of one disease implied over twice the chance of having a second of a different type.

Behavioural impairment

The great majority of these retarded children also suffered from some form of behaviour disturbance. Of a larger sample of 142 normal-appearing retarded children, of whom the above 102 were the most severely affected, only 24·5 per cent were of stable temperament;

42 per cent were unforthcoming, 18·1 were unstable or hyperactive, and 15·5 suffered from other types of maladjustment. Among mentally normal children, between 60 and 75 per cent, according to the nature of the sample, may be reckoned as stable. The tendency to multiple impairment seems, therefore, to extend to behaviour disturbance.

Possible causative factors

Among the group of retarded children the predominant type of behaviour disturbance, unforthcomingness, is a clearly defined condition, so that its relationship to possible causative factors can be tested. Within this specialized sample of handicapped children it bore no relation to severe early ill health ($\chi^2 = 0{\cdot}14$), although in a heterogeneous sample including a wide range of mental ability it would probably do so, since retarded children are more likely both to be unforthcoming and to have a history of early illness. The lack of a relation within this sample, however, suggests that there is no direct connection between the two: it seems improbable that the illnesses themselves caused damage to the nervous structures controlling motivation.

Unforthcoming children are unventuresome and timid, so that they are observed to be very dependent upon their mothers. This has led some psychologists to suppose that their overdependence has been brought about by anxious, over-solicitous mothers who have always done everything for their children and robbed them of initiative. To test this possibility over the sample of retarded children, the mothers' personalities were classified into three broad groups: stable, anxious, and unstable/inadequate. The unforthcoming children were found to be distributed fairly evenly among all three: the stable mothers had only slightly fewer than their due share (19, with a statistical expectation of 22·8), and the other two groups only slightly more[59] (the anxious having 11, with an expectation of 9; and the unstable/inadequate 14, with an expectation of 12·1). Overdependence, as an aspect of unforthcomingness, does not seem therefore to be a reflection of maternal personality. More likely, the appearance of overprotection was produced by the care that these, on the whole normally affectionate, mothers gave to children who were not ready for independence.

Unforthcomingness was similarly unrelated to separation from the mother during the first three years, proportionately fewer of the unforthcoming children (25·4 per cent) having been separated than of the stable or the unsettled/maladjusted (34·3 and 33·3 per cent respectively). Once again, owing to the tendency to multiple impairment, an association between unforthcomingness and separation (in the form of hospitalization) is likely to be found in a heterogeneous sample. But the condition is evidently not caused by the separation itself.

As a final test of possible postnatal environmental influence, the children's families were classified according to abnormal structure (illegitimacy, broken home, long separation, etc.) and insecurity-producing relationships between child and parent. These were amalgamated into one broad category of abnormal family situation. The proportion of unforthcoming children in this category (41·3 per cent) was almost precisely equal to that (41·7 per cent) among children in normal family situations. It seems unlikely, in consequence, that unforthcomingness is a form of reaction to familial insecurity.

On the other hand, a clear relation emerged between this type of personality defect and illness or other stress to the mother during the pregnancy ($\chi^2 = 10{\cdot}17$, $n = 1$, $p < {\cdot}01$ and approaching ·001). Moreover, there was a significant tendency for it to be related to stresses during the later part of pregnancy. It is probably at this stage that the fine mechanisms that control behaviour develop. Unforthcomingness could thus be caused by congenital damage to the nervous system. This would account for its prevalence among the mentally retarded and (as will be seen below) among unhealthy children within a normal population.

Multiple Impairment and Infant Hospitalization

The sample of mentally retarded children presented an intricate complex of early ill health, behaviour disturbance, and separation, in which it was difficult to untangle the causal relationships. It was therefore necessary to start from a different angle, by studying a sample of children who had been ill in infancy.[60] From the records of the Royal Hospital for Sick Children at Bristol were selected all those who, during 1946 and 1947, had been retained at least two weeks during their first two years of life. Owing to the difficulty of tracing them after several years, those whose homes were outside the city's boundary were excluded, as also were illegitimate and foster children and those who had subsequently died. Of the net sample of 198 it was possible to find 142, or 72 per cent, in 1955, when the children were between seven and eleven years of age. Since there was a separate hospital in the city for infectious diseases all the conditions for which they had been treated in the Royal Hospital as infants were of a non-epidemic character. The diagnoses were taken as entered in the hospital records. Though some of these may have been inaccurate, they were at least made independently of the children's subsequent mental and emotional development, except for two infants who had been admitted because of suspected mental deficiency.

Controls of the same sex and birth-date were taken from the schools attended by the early-hospital children, except that no controls were chosen to match those who were in special schools since this would have introduced a systematic bias. Thus the 133 controls constituted a reasonably random sample, among whom some would have been ill or in hospital as infants.

Attainment in reading

The teachers were asked to rate attainment in reading and arithmetic on a five-point scale. Since the results for both subjects were similar, only those for reading are quoted (*Table 20*). The early-hospital

Table 20 Early-hospital children: attainment in reading

	N	*Definitely retarded*	*Slightly retarded*	*Average or superior*
		%	%	%
Early-hospital children	142	27·5	27·5	45·0
Controls	133	11·3	21·8	67·0

group were more retarded in reading, at a risk of chance of less than 1 in a 1000 ($\chi^2 = 15{\cdot}0$, $n = 2$). Their degree of retardation was unrelated to their length of stay in hospital; in effect, fewer of the very backward had had long spells in hospital – of eight weeks or more – than of the average or superior readers (7·7 compared with 12·7 per cent).[70] Thus it is improbable that the greater degree of backwardness among the early-hospital children was due to their hospital experience or to the separation from the mother that it entailed.

There remained the possibility that the association between infantile illness and reading backwardness was produced by a social-class bias: the poorer working-class children might have had more illness or, because of lack of facilities for nursing at home, might have been sent to hospital more readily. All the homes were visited and assessed upon a socio-economic five-point scale. None of the eight middle-class children was backward in reading, six of them being in fact superior; in contrast, eight of the ten poorer working-class children were backward and none was superior. Among the 96 children who came in the general working-class group, however, with adequate standards of housekeeping and hygiene, the greater extent of reading backwardness compared with the controls was even more pronounced than it was in the undifferentiated total sample. The proportion of definitely retarded rose from 27·5 to 30·2 per cent; furthermore, the proportion of average or superior readers fell from 45 to 38·5 per cent. The effect of removing the extreme socio-economic groups was to render the association between infantile illness and reading backwardness closer still ($\chi^2 = 20{\cdot}5$, $n = 2$, $p < {\cdot}001$).

Behaviour disturbance

The teachers completed the Bristol Social Adjustment Guides for the early-hospital children and their controls, with results as shown in *Table 21*. There are actually slightly more unsettled and maladjusted

Table 21 Early-hospital children: incidence of behaviour disturbance

	Stable	*Unforthcoming*	*Unsettled*	*Maladjusted*	*Total*
Early-hospital children	45	66	17	9	137
%	(33)	(48)	(12)	(7)	
Controls	52	46	24	8	130
%	(40)	(35)	(19)	(6)	

children among the controls – apart from the unforthcoming – than among the hospital children; but the excess of unforthcomingness among the latter is significant at the ·05 level. Once again a statistical association is found between this personality defect and early illness; but it means only that the same children tend both to be ill in infancy and to be unforthcoming in mid-childhood. The earlier study of mentally retarded children had indicated that there was probably no direct causal connection between unforthcomingness and early illness.

Effects of early illness

To summarize, the study of hospital children revealed a nexus of intercorrelation between severe infantile illness, a characteristic childhood defect of temperament, and backwardness in reading and arithmetic. The question to be decided was whether any of the three major handicaps – in health, temperament, or ability – was primary, or whether all were the results of some common causative factor.

It had first to be ascertained whether the multiple handicaps could be traced to any particular illness or group of illnesses. The first conditions to come under suspicion were those that might have been the direct cause of brain damage. The early-hospital group included fifteen cases of meningitis, encephalitis, congenital syphilis, or poliomyelitis, but seven of the children concerned were average or forward readers. The infantile disease most closely associated with reading backwardness was pneumonia: of the twenty-one cases, twelve were severely or definitely retarded, five mildly so, and only four were average or superior readers. Even when these cases were excluded, however, the hospital children were still more backward than the controls at a risk of chance of about 1 in 100 ($\chi^2 = 9{\cdot}0$, $n = 2$). The relationship, in short, was with infantile illness in general rather than with a particular illness.

This still left open the question whether the early illnesses were responsible for the defects of temperament and poor school attainment, or whether they were the co-results of a shared cause. So far as is at present known, the only way in which childhood illness can have such after-effects, apart from direct infection of brain tissue, is through acute fever. A single case of poliomyelitis was the only viral infection. Among the remaining illnesses for which the children were admitted very few would have been accompanied by fever so acute as to produce neural damage. It was improbable, therefore, that the scholastic retardation and unforthcomingness were the direct outcome of the illnesses.

Evidence for a Congenital Common Factor

It is when we come to explore the possibility of a common, congenital cause that the evidence is strongest and most consistent. Among 188 cases of mental retardation, including the 142 referred to above, and their 450 mentally normal controls, non-epidemic infantile illness was approximately three times more frequent following physical illness or mental stress during the pregnancy (for the retarded, $\chi^2 = 31{\cdot}4$, $p < {\cdot}001$; for the normal, $\chi^2 = 30{\cdot}6$, $p < {\cdot}001$).[57, 70] The very closeness of this relationship suggests a direct causal connection. Moreover, the personality defect in question, and such malformations as were observed, were associated with the same disturbances of pregnancy. A similar deficiency of motivation has been experimentally produced in rats[2, 78] and in mice[33] by subjecting the pregnant animals to stress.

The series of interrelationships is given meaning by a concept of multiple congenital impairment. This may be formulated in the following proposition: if a child suffers from one sort of handicap – physical, mental, or temperamental – there is an increased risk of his being affected in some other way in addition. If, for example, the child has one sort of physical weakness resulting in disease, there will be a greater likelihood of disease of another type, or of mental retardation, or of disorder of motivation. Conversely, if mental retardation is observed, there is a greater likelihood of physical illness and/or of behaviour disturbance. The rationale of this phenomenon is that congenital damage tends to affect the child in more than one way, and this is especially so when the central nervous system is the seat of the trauma. It follows as corollary that if two or more distinct types of ill health are observed in a child the probability of their having a congenital origin is greater, and hence there is a greater chance of mental or emotional handicap.

It was possible to put this deduction to the test by reference to the data of the early-hospital study. The children were divided into two groups, those who had had only a single type of disorder and those who had had two or more distinct types. With the help of a paediatrician on the staff of the hospital the diagnoses as given in the records were divided into four classes: respiratory disease; digestive disease; local infection; other reason for admission (in most cases this was the treatment of congenital defects). Illnesses were rated as distinct if they fell into different categories; but two in the fourth group were also accounted such if they affected different parts of the body and did not belong to any known syndrome. Of the 102 infants treated for one disorder only, 47 per cent were subsequently backward readers; of the 37 treated for two or more disorders the proportion was as high as 73 per cent, this being significant at less than the ·01 level ($\chi^2 = 7{\cdot}26$, $n = 1$).

The presence of more than one type of disease in a child seems to indicate, therefore, the greatest likelihood of multiple congenital impairment. Some of those admitted to hospital with only one disease would have been normally robust children who had been exposed to heavy infection. This would apply in particular to the digestive cases owing to the risk of enteritic infection in infancy. Where, on the other hand, the disease of the digestive system is accompanied by another disorder there is more reason to suspect a congenital origin, and the hypothesis would predict a relatively greater excess of backwardness in those cases. This was in fact so: only 41 per cent of the digestive-only cases suffered any degree of reading retardation compared with no less than 82 per cent of those with a digestive condition plus one or more other types of disease.

Hypothesis of Cumulative Impairment

This confirmation of a tendency to cumulative impairment enables us to state the hypothesis more formally in the following terms: if a child suffers from one form of somatic-neural impairment there is a greater than chance probability that he will be affected by a second; if he suffers from two, there is a still greater chance of a third, and so on in geometrical progression until the point of non-viability is reached.

The crucial test of a hypothesis is its predictive value in relation to different samples. Our present one would predict, for example, that, in general, maladjusted children would show a greater incidence of physical illness and defect than would non-maladjusted children.

Evidence from a Sample of Delinquent Boys

In the Glasgow study of all delinquent boys put on probation for the first time in 1957, a very high proportion were maladjusted compared with non-delinquent controls in the same schools, born on the same dates or the dates nearest to these.[61] The delinquents and controls combined thus provided a convenient sample containing a good representation of all degrees of behaviour disturbance.

Maladjustment and physical impairment

The types of ill health and physical defect found among them were divided into five categories, as in *Table 22*. Physical defects covered squint, bad hearing, poor muscular coordination and spastic tendencies, speech defect, and congenital malformation. Abnormality of growth included all boys rated by their teachers as diminutive, very fat, or very thin. No boy was counted more than once in any category even though he might have qualified by more than one physical impairment.[67]

Table 22 Probationers and controls: maladjustment and physical impairment

Physical impairment	*BSAG score categories* 0–4	5–9	10–19	20+	χ^2*	*p*
	N=231	*N*=157	*N*=213	*N*=217		
	%	%	%	%		
Respiratory disease	9·1	16·1	18·8	31·3	36·60	>·001
Other ailments	5·6	11·5	13·2	25·4	37·53	>·001
Physical defects	3·5	6·4	7·5	14·3	18·96	>·001
Growth abnormality	4·3	6·4	11·7	14·8	14·25	>·001
Poor eyesight	5·2	10·8	10·3	14·3	10·46	>·01

* Two degrees of freedom; the two central score categories are combined

It is seen from *Table 22* and *Figure 2*, which presents the same data in a histogram, that the incidence of all the types of ill health or defect rises consistently with the degree of behaviour disturbance, at a very high level of significance. The tendency was equally apparent among the probationers and the controls, but among the former it was possible to ascertain to what degree, if any, these associations between maladjustment and physical impairment could be the result of a common factor of inadequate living conditions or a disorganized cultural background.

The cultural assessment was based on that of Jephcott and Carter.[30] The families were classified, by means of a Cultural-Group Schedule,[68] in four groups as follows:

I. Standard conscious and socially aspiring
II. 'Respectable' working-class standards but not aspiring to those of the middle class
III. 'Getting along' on a low standard
IV. Not 'getting along': home unkempt and dirty, and family life disorganized.

Of the 414 probationer-delinquents' families, 231 could be clearly apportioned to 'adequate' cultural groups (I and II). The association

Figure 2 PROBATIONERS AND CONTROLS: MALADJUSTMENT AND PHYSICAL IMPAIRMENT

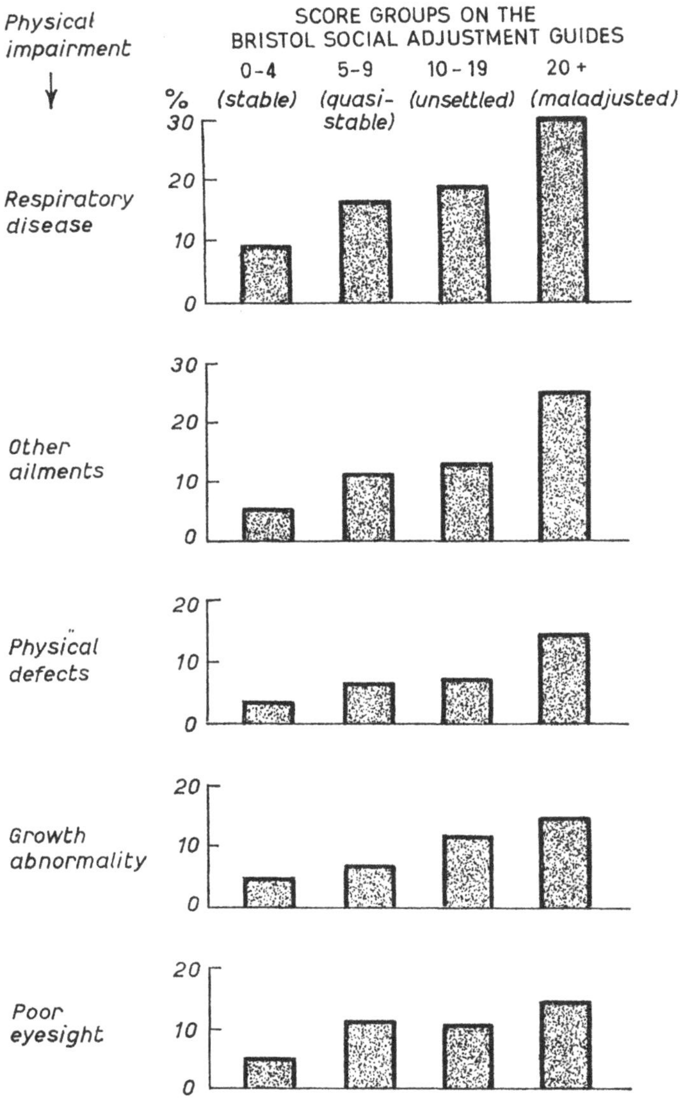

between maladjustment and physical impairment was then tested within these two groups alone. The results, summarized in the last column of *Table 23*, show that over twice as many of the disturbed delinquents (those with 10 or more indications of maladjustment) suffered from respiratory disease, and similar proportions from other ailments and growth abnormality.

Table 23 Probationers from homes of adequate standard: maladjustment and physical impairment

Physical impairment	BSAG score categories 0–9	10–19	20+	Ratio* %(10+) / %(0–9)
	N=62	N=77	N=92	
	%	%	%	
Respiratory disease	9·7	19·5	23·9	2·26
Other ailments	8·1	15·5	17·4	2·06
Physical defects	1·6	5·2	6·5	3·68
Growth abnormality	6·4	9·1	17·4	2·12
Poor eyesight	4·8	7·8	10·9	1·96

* The proportionately greater incidence of each physical condition among probationers scoring 10 or more compared with those scoring 9 or less.

In *Figure 3* the data in *Table 23* for probationers from adequate homes are compared with those for all probationers irrespective of cultural level. It is seen that inadequate family standards are responsible for only a small part of the association between behaviour disturbance and ill health. In an earlier study of Glasgow delinquents,[16] Ferguson found, as expected, that the number of undersized boys among his delinquent sample was significantly greater than the number among his controls. He assumed that this was due to the fact that a greater proportion of delinquents belong to underprivileged social groups. Nevertheless, he found that the association between delinquency and small stature held good even for those delinquents coming from homes of a good standard, and he could offer no explanation for it.

These consistent intercorrelations between physical impairment and behaviour disturbance are open to interpretation on Adlerian lines, in the sense that the boys may have compensated for their physical inferiorities by misbehaviour. The nearest approach to inferiority compensation would be recorded in the Bristol Guides in the XC syndrome (anxiety for approval of and acceptance by age

Figure 3 PROBATIONERS: MALADJUSTMENT AND PHYSICAL IMPAIRMENT RELATED TO HOME CONDITIONS

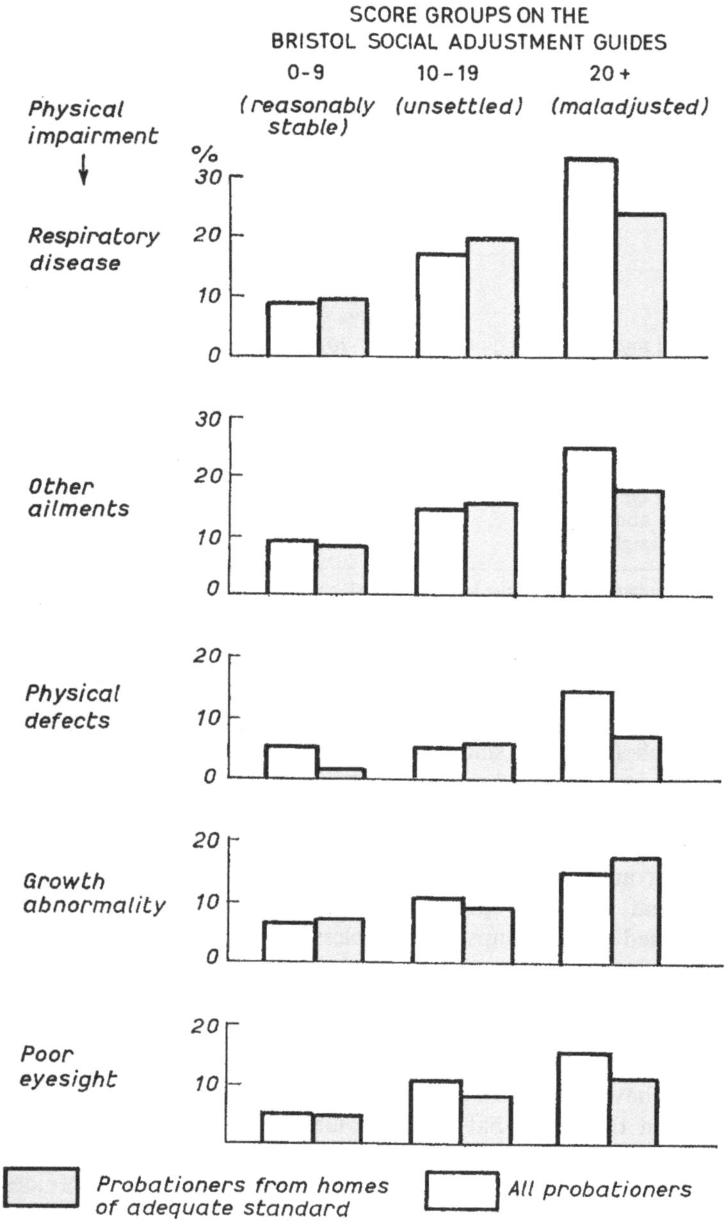

peers), typical items in which are: 'Can't resist playing to the crowd'; 'Brags to other children'; 'Damage to public property'; 'Foolish pranks when with a gang'. This syndrome accounted for only 15 of the total of 166 scored items of disturbed behaviour. Moreover, it proved to be less associated with ill health than did other types of behaviour disturbance: the proportion of unhealthy boys having a significant XC score (24·1 per cent) was lower than the mean incidence (31·0 per cent) for other syndromes.

The multiple-disease test

In the absence, therefore, of any known alternative explanation in terms of social conditions or inferiority compensation, the tendency for maladjusted boys to be unhealthy or otherwise physically impaired must be taken as confirming the hypothesis of multiple congenital impairment. It remained to test the latter further, in the same group of delinquents and controls, by the multiple-disease corollary. This would predict that boys with two distinct diseases would be more prone to behaviour disturbance than would those with only one or no disease. *Table 24* shows that this tendency is confirmed among both the delinquents and the controls, but more strikingly among the former. Only about half as many of the maladjusted were healthy compared with the stable, and thirteen times as many of them were in the multiple-disease category. Of the 71 in this category, only five were reasonably stable.

It is of interest to note that among the controls the proportion of boys affected by multiple disease remains fairly constant for all categories above a BSAG score of 5, whereas it is small (2·7 per cent) among the stable. Among the delinquents multiple disease does not rise sharply until a score of 20 is passed. The explanation could be that boys who show evidence of multiple disease are vulnerable to environmental stresses, but their vulnerability manifests itself in severe behaviour disturbance only when – as presumably among the delinquents – they are exposed to insecure or otherwise stressful family situations. Boys with a similar degree of vulnerability in good family situations would show only mild disturbance and little delinquency.

Despite the great disparities between the mean BSAG scores for the delinquents and the controls, the mean scores for the multiple-disease boys in both groups are significantly higher than those for boys with only one disease. A proportion of the single diseases occurring in otherwise healthy boys would no doubt be due to exposure

Table 24 Probationers and controls: maladjustment and multiple disease

	N	*BSAG score categories* 0–4	5–9	10–19	20+	*Mean score*	*t and p for differences of adjacent means*
PROBATIONERS		%	%	%	%		
No disease	234	82·2	73·6	60·2	43·1	16·39	
							2·676 <·01
One disease only	109	15·6	18·9	30·5	28·2	19·71	
							4·483 <·001
Two or more distinct diseases	71	2·2	7·6	9·4	28·7	26·90	
CONTROLS							
No disease	276	78·5	57·7	65·9	48·3	6·45	
							1·545 n.s.
One disease only	79	18·8	21·2	15·3	31·0	8·05	
							2·131
Two or more distinct diseases	49	2·7	21·2	18·8	20·7	11·04	·05

to infection or to adverse living conditions. On the other hand, the presence of two or more distinct diseases would confer a greater probability of congenital impairment, as seen in the above early-hospital children. It is noteworthy that, among both delinquents and controls, the differences in the mean scores are greater between the one-disease and the multiple-disease groups than between the no-disease and the one-disease groups. This finding confirms the cumulative aspect of multiple impairment: the more a child has, the more he is likely to have.

Health of delinquents

The Glasgow delinquency study afforded a further opportunity for testing the hypothesis that a predisposition to behaviour disturbance forms part of a syndrome of multiple congenital impairment. Because of other important factors that determine whether a boy becomes delinquent or not – his cultural, family, and school environments; whether he is caught; and, if caught, whether he is charged – we cannot expect a high relationship between delinquency and congenital impairment. Nevertheless delinquency is a form of abnormal behaviour in the widest sense. (No known social group permits stealing from its own members or social deviance that embroils it with society at large.) The youthful delinquent tends to show characteristic forms of other behaviour disturbance. The hypothesis of multiple impairment would thus predict that delinquents would be more prone to ill health and physical defect than non-delinquents. The Gluecks[20] found no such tendency, but it must be remembered that they took their sample of delinquents from those who had been committed to correctional schools. Apart from the fact that it is necessary to be certified as medically fit for this kind of treatment, the sample would probably be further biased in the direction of robustness by the decision of the court: a healthy aggressive-looking young fellow is more likely to be committed for correctional training than a puny, unhealthy-looking one. The sample of Glasgow probationers were somewhat more unhealthy on the average than the non-delinquent controls – 38 per cent more of them having respiratory diseases and 78 per cent more having one or more other ailments ($p < \cdot 05$ and $< \cdot 02$ respectively).[68]

A more critical test of a congenital factor in delinquency would be to ascertain whether the delinquents had suffered an excessive amount of ill health in early infancy. It was consequently decided to consult the Health Visitors' records of the health of the Glasgow probationers during their first twelve months of life. Unfortunately, by the time this decision was made, the cards for the older age-groups had already been destroyed (on their attaining the age of fifteen years) and it was therefore possible to consult only the records for those, numbering 136, who had appeared in court between the ages of eight and eleven years. To serve as controls, the records were examined of the two boy babies born nearest in time to each of the delinquent sample, and in the same street or similar social surroundings. The effect of this matching was to equalize, so far as could be, the cultural and socio-economic background of the infants who became delinquents with that of infants whose subsequent history was unknown. A significantly greater number of the records of the future delinquents contained one or more adverse health comments ($\chi^2 = 3\cdot435$, $p < \cdot 05$ on a one-tailed hypothesis). Many of these comments, however, referred to quite minor disorders, so a record of the infant's having been taken into hospital was taken as an

Table 25 Probationers and controls: hospitalization in infancy

	N	*Admitted to hospital in first year of life*	*No record of hospital admittance*
Probationers	136	16 (11·8%)	120
Controls	272	10 (3·7%)	262

$\chi^2 = 9{\cdot}93$ ($p < {\cdot}005$ on a one-tailed hypothesis)

objective criterion of more serious illness. The findings, which are given in *Table 25*, are highly significant and in the predicted direction.

The higher hospitalization rate in infancy of the delinquent group was unlikely to have resulted from a greater readiness on the part of their doctors to secure admittance for them on account of the low standard of their homes, since the Health Visitors rated only four of the latter as dirty or untidy.

Once again, the multiple-disease test indicated a congenital origin for the infantile-disease proneness of those who were subsequently delinquent. It was seen from *Table 24* that a really significant increase in behaviour disturbance was found in those children who had two or more diseases of different types, as compared with those who were healthy or had only one type. The same increase was noted in relation to the infantile health of the delinquents: there was no significant difference in the subsequent social adjustment of those who had had no disease or only one, and their mean BSAG score, between the ages of eight and eleven years, was 16·9; for the eleven who had a record of multiple disease, the mean was 29·2. This tendency was even more marked in the Delinquency Prediction scores: the mean for the one-or-none group was 20·7, whereas that for the multiple-disease group was 46·6.

It was unlikely, however, that the delinquency was due to the early hospitalization. A greater proportion of the delinquent group had been unhealthy as infants apart from those who went into hospital. In addition, if the hospitalization had had any such dramatic long-term effect it would probably have been reflected in the severity of their general behaviour disturbance; in fact, those hospitalized were slightly less disturbed (BSAG score 15·25) than the non-hospitalized (18·47). The relatively larger number of delinquents who had been admitted to hospital in infancy could be accounted for by the greater severity of their illnesses, and this would have been predicted by the multiple-impairment hypothesis.

Multiple Impairment in a Normal Sample

The all-British truancy survey described in Chapter Seven afforded a further opportunity for confirming the tendency to multiple impairment among boys and for testing it among girls. The reader is reminded that the control children consisted of two groups, those born on the same day as the truants or the nearest day, and those born in the same year and living in the same or nearest street. Since the same trend was apparent in both control groups they are amalgamated in *Table 26*.

Table 26 Mean BSAG scores of healthy and unhealthy children: controls of truants, aged 7–15 years

Physical condition	*N*	*Boys*	*N*	*Girls*
With respiratory disease	59	12·19	14	15·71
No respiratory disease	371	7·29	155	5·97
Critical ratio		4·115		3·746
p		<·001		<·001
With other ailment	37	14·03	18	15·17
With no other ailment	393	7·36	151	5·63
Critical ratio		3·500		4·264
p		<·001		<·001

Whether they suffer from respiratory or other disease, unhealthy children are in general significantly more disturbed than healthy, at a consistent risk of chance of less than 1 in 1,000.

Truants: Maladjustment and Ill Health

It is interesting that there was comparatively little difference as regards severity of behaviour disturbance between healthy and unhealthy truants. The mean BSAG scores for the latter were consistently higher, but the difference reached significance only for the girl truants in respect of respiratory disease (*Table 27*).

This result suggests that most truants come within the class of children who have suffered congenital damage, so that other signs of

Table 27 Mean BSAG scores of healthy and unhealthy truants

Physical condition	*N*	*Boys*	*N*	*Girls*
With respiratory disease	52	26·73	13	29·69
No respiratory disease	168	24·37	72	23·14
Critical ratio		1·192		2·229
p		n.s.		>·05
With other ailment	46	25·97	18	24·72
With no other ailment	174	24·77	67	23·98
Critical ratio		0·603		0·234
p		n.s.		n.s.

the latter, such as a tendency to ill health, will not discriminate well between them. This does not mean that most of the truants were actually unhealthy, although twice as many of them suffered from respiratory disease and over twice as many from other diseases, compared with the controls. It must be emphasized that multiple impairment is a tendency only. By no means all the impaired children would be affected in health as well as in personality. Thus there would be a proportion who would be healthy, yet with a kind of neural dysfunction that renders them prone to behaviour disturbance. The extremely high mean BSAG scores for the truants (24·93 for the boys and 24·14 for the girls, *Tables 7* and *8* above) support this explanation.

Sex Differences as Evidence of Congenitality

The probability that the complex of diverse impairments that we are studying has a congenital origin is strengthened by the observation of consistent sex differences. These are of a twofold character. The first is that boys are more prone than girls to every type of handicap (except malformation of the central nervous system). The second is that, provided the handicap is of a type that permits of recovery, affected boys show a better recovery rate than girls. Morrison Smith's study of asthma in schoolchildren[53] illustrates both these apparently contradictory tendencies (*Table 28*).

Table 28 Prevalence of asthma among Birmingham schoolchildren

Ages	*Boys*	*Girls*
5 and 6	227 (2·58%)	82 (1·02%)
10 and 11	202 (2·33%)	101 (1·29%)
13, 14, and 15	152 (1·96%)	101 (1·21%)

Source: Morrison J. Smith (1961)[53]

In boys the incidence is seen to fall by about 32 per cent between the ages of five and fifteen. In girls it rises by some 20 per cent, but the increase is probably due to the greater chance of a diagnosis having been made by the time children reach the ages of thirteen to fifteen years. For the same reason, the extent of the improvement in boys is probably understated. The effect of the contradictory trends is that in the youngest age-group asthma is 150 per cent more prevalent among boys as compared with girls, but only 25 per cent more so in the oldest age-group.

A congenital basis for asthma

It is of course not universally agreed that asthma is a congenital impairment. The observation that the condition is aggravated by emotional stress has led to the assumption that it is 'psychogenic'. Taken literally, this term implies that in some otherwise normal children emotional stress produces asthma. But the vast majority of children do not react thus to emotional stress, so that there must be some initial susceptibility. In fact, other conditions – epilepsy, speech defect, squint – can similarly be aggravated by stress, and no one doubts that in them the root cause is a neurological impairment which is nearly always congenital. Such variations may be described as the outcome of an interaction between an initial predisposition and postnatal stress. There is a further reason for inferring a congenital origin to asthma. As has been pointed out, the probability that a condition is congenital is higher – barring a demonstrable environmental connection – if it is found in association with other impairments. The probability is even greater if these are observed in early infancy, before environmental stresses have had time to be effective.

In an intensive study of twenty-five asthmatics, matched with twenty-five controls of similar sex, socio-economic status, position in family, and amount of childhood illness, Burton[7] found that the asthmatics were significantly more disturbed in their behaviour during their first two years of life (*Table 29*). Eleven of the mothers of the asthmatics stated that they had been subjected to emotionally upsetting circumstances or other complication during the pregnancy (illegitimacy, bad housing, death in the family, threatened miscarriage, anaemia, excessive sickness, toxaemia, etc.), whereas only two of the mothers of the non-asthmatics were similarly affected.

Table 29 Asthma and behaviour problems in infancy

Incidence of behaviour problems (excessive crying, poor feeding, vomiting, etc.)	*Asthmatics*	*Non-asthmatics*	*Significance*
First year	13	6	·046
Second year	9	1	·02

Source: L. Burton (1964)[7]

At the time when they were the subject of investigation, during their school years, the asthmatics were only moderately more disturbed than the controls (BSAG scores of 8·46 and 6·25 respectively), but it must be remembered that the controls also had had more than the normal amount of childhood illness owing to the method of matching used. When the six chronically ill controls were excluded the remaining nineteen had a mean score of only 4·7. The most significant behavioural characteristic of the asthmatics was their greater degree of unforthcomingness ($p = {\cdot}008$); next to this was a tendency to withdrawal ($p = {\cdot}023$) and indifference to social attachments (K-type behaviour) ($p = {\cdot}045$). There is reason to believe that these varieties of personality defect have a congenital basis.

Greater incidence of physical and emotional impairment in boys

The existence of a consistent sex difference in the incidence of impairment is hard to explain except in genetic terms. A greater incidence among males is found for many childhood illnesses. Drillien[15] found that premature boys had 20–30 per cent more respiratory disease for all grades of maternal care. In Scotland as a whole pneumonia is 35 per cent more frequent in boys than in girls under five years of age, and eight times as many of the boys die from this disease.[52] Among the 450 mentally normal controls of the mentally retarded sample studied by the writer[57] nearly twice as many boys as girls had suffered serious non-epidemic illness in their first three years (22·8 per cent of the boys, 12·2 of the girls).

An interesting sidelight on the greater susceptibility of boys to ill health is provided in Wilson's study[79] of children in 'performance-inadequate' (culturally disintegrated) families. In order to equalize the cultural and material environment she chose as controls a number of families of similar size living in the same streets or closes. One of the most tell-tale aspects of the comparison is that there are 22·6 per cent more girls in the performance-inadequate families – the details of which are given in *Table 30*. Among the controls there were actually

Table 30 Sex distribution in culturally disintegrated families

	Boys	*Girls*
Culturally disintegrated families	517	634
Control families	663	622

Source: Wilson (1962)[79] $\chi^2 = 10{\cdot}82$, $p = {\cdot}001$

6·6 per cent more boys, which is rather more than the usual excess of males born. The latter is due to the greater liability of female embryos to malformation of the central nervous system, and since this occurs during the first month after conception a certain number of embryonic deaths, preponderantly female, take place without the pregnancy having been recognized. That there were at least 6 per cent fewer girls born suggests that even the control families were living under stressful conditions, and it is likely that in the performance-inadequate families there was a similar excess of boys born. This would mean an excess childhood loss of approximately 29 per cent for the boys. It is reasonable to assume that those who survived would nevertheless have been more than usually subject to the sorts of congenital impairment that do not carry the hazard of premature death. Among these, behaviour disturbance would figure largely. Accordingly, the very high incidence of delinquency that Wilson observed among the children from performance-inadequate families cannot be attributed entirely to neglect.

The incidence of common habit disorders shows similar sex differences. Among Drillien's sample of premature children 15 per cent of the boys but only 7 per cent of the girls were still wet at night at five years. Douglas and Mulligan[14] likewise found much less bedwetting among girls during middle childhood.

Since they provide a score based on a large number of indications of behaviour disturbance the Bristol Social Adjustment Guides are able to show more general sex differences. The overall picture resembles that for asthma, the boys being more affected but showing a better recovery rate. In industrial centres in South Wales Chazan[9] found that at the primary stage – up to eleven years – only 50 per cent of the boys compared with 69 per cent of the girls fell in the 'very stable' category (scores of 0–4); at the secondary stages – eleven to fifteen years – the proportion of well-adjusted girls remained the same, but the boys had improved to 62·5 per cent. Among the controls of the all-British survey of truants the percentage of boys in the very stable category similarly improved – from 42·8 to 46·0; by contrast, that for the girls deteriorated from 58·6 to 51·4. It will be noted, however, that the girls were better adjusted than the boys at all ages. This result was unlikely to be due to a sex bias in the Bristol Guides, since girls who pick themselves out by some index form of aberrant behaviour such as delinquency or truancy score just as highly on average as the corresponding types of boys.

Virtually all non-lethal congenital malformations are more frequent among boys. The same applies to mental deficiency, including mongolism, and educational subnormality. In a study of IQ changes on retest among a sample of mentally subnormal children, involving 952 such children and 1,358 comparisons,[63] boys did relatively better than girls at the retest between one and four years later, at a significance level of less than 1 in 1,000. Present indications are that girls show much less motor impairment than boys. Consistent with the general picture, however, boys seem to recover partially or completely from moderate motor impairment following puberty, but insufficient work has been done in this field to yield systematic findings.

Multiple Impairment: A Congenital Basis

Implications of the term 'congenital'

We have now to review what direct evidence there is for believing that multiple impairment has mainly a congenital origin. To obviate misunderstanding the reader should be reminded at this stage that the word 'congenital' is used in the strict sense that the condition originates at or before birth. It need not be actually observable at birth, and the defect may take the form of a predisposition which is actualized only by some postnatal factor. For example, epileptic fits that first appear in mid-childhood may be described as congenital if they are the result of neural damage at birth, and the same applies to many infantile illnesses which are more frequent following a disturbed pregnancy. The mistake is often committed of referring to influences acting postnatally as 'environmental' and the rest as 'hereditary'. But those acting prenatally can also be environmental, and seem in fact mostly to be so. For this reason 'congenital' is the more exact term, and the one less likely to lead us into error. Naturally, since genetic factors are present prior to birth, they are included in the term congenital. More will be said later about the interaction of genetic and environmental factors during gestation.

Congenitally conferred vulnerability

Congenital damage most often takes the form of a disposition to breakdown or malfunction. The affected child is rendered more vulnerable to stress. There is consequently also an interaction, in the period following birth, between congenital impairment and adverse environmental influences.

This is convincingly demonstrated by Drillien[15] in her intensive

Table 31 Intelligence-test scores of premature and mature-born children by birth weight and social grade

Birth weight	*Social grade* *Superior working class or higher*	*Average working class*	*Poor working class*
Prematurely born children			
up to 3½ lbs	93	82	77
over 3½ to 4½ lbs	108	95	90
over 4½ to 5½ lbs	110	101	90
Mature-born children			
over 5½ lbs	114	102	98
Difference between scores of small prematures and mature-born	21	20	21

Source: Drillien(1964)[15]

follow-up study of a large sample of prematurely born children. She divided them and the mature-born controls into three social groups corresponding to those used in the early-hospital study. *Table 31* shows the mean Terman-Merrill intelligence-test scores of the children at 5–7 years, by birth weight and social grade. The smaller the birth weight the lower, on average, the IQ, irrespective of social grade; and the differences between the small prematures and the mature-born (over 5½ lbs) are remarkably constant at 20–21 points. However, adverse living conditions and deficiency of intellectual stimulation within the poor working-class and, to a lesser extent, the average working-class groups likewise produce a depression of the test results.

The effect of adverse living conditions was even more pronounced in social adjustment. Underprivileged social status brings with it a higher degree of family insecurity and other stress, especially when it is associated – as tends to be the case – with an element of social disintegration. *Table 32* gives the percentages of maladjusted children (BSAG score of 20 or over) at seven years, by birth weight and social grade. Irrespective of social class the small premature children show more maladjustment at seven years, but the greater stress associated with an underprivileged environment magnifies the initial vulnerability.

The cumulative effect of congenital damage and of adverse post-natal environment is even more strikingly illustrated in *Table 33*. Examination of the table shows that the presence of pregnancy/delivery complications alone increases the mean scores of both the premature and the mature groups by about 65 per cent. Family stresses alone seem to affect the premature children more severely than the mature-born. Where, however, family stresses are added to pregnancy/delivery complications the mean for the prematures tops the maladjusted mark, and the mature-born also score highly. Drillien's comment is worth quoting:

> 'It is of particular interest, in view of current theories stressing the importance of maternal handling and early experience, to note that three-quarters of those mature controls who were subjected to severe familial stress in their early years appeared to be emotionally stable (at 7 years), and less than 1 in 10 showed borderline to obvious maladjustment, but this proportion rose to nearly one-half where there had been complications before or during birth and to over one-half when, in addition, birth weight was 4½ lbs or less.'

To sum up the findings of this important work of Drillien, the congenital handicaps do not *in themselves* produce a high degree of behaviour disturbance at seven years. They render the child more vulnerable to postnatal stresses. It should be emphasized that this finding is not confined to premature children, for the same additive tendency is seen among the mature controls.

Table 32 Behaviour disturbance among premature and mature-born children by birth weight and social grade

	Social grade		
Birth weight	*Superior working class or higher*	*Average working class*	*Poor working class*
	Percentage with BSAG score of 20 or over		
Prematurely born children			
4½ lbs and under	10·4	25·0	51·4
4½ to 5½ lbs	5·0	4·0	27·0
Mature-born children			
over 5½ lbs	6·1	5·9	31·3

Source: Drillien (1964)[15]

Table 33 Congenital and postnatal determinants of behaviour disturbance

	Mean BSAG scores for	
	Small prematures (4½ lbs or less)	*Mature-born (over 5½ lbs)*
No pregnancy/ delivery complications; no family stress	6·4	4·9
Pregnancy/delivery complications; no family stress	10·5	8·2
Family stress; no pregnancy/delivery complications	13·1	7·5
Pregnancy/delivery complications; family stress	20·0	15·6

Source: Drillien (1964)[15]

Facilitation by gestational stress

The preponderance of impairment among males points to some form of genetic sex-linkage. Nevertheless, though a slight hereditary tendency is found in all the common non-epidemic childhood illnesses (Marshall, Hutchinson & Honisett [38a]), it never approaches a Mendelian regularity. We have to look, therefore, for some special kind of genetic influence. Analogous animal studies suggest that it takes the form of a potentiality for defect which – to use the term proposed by Malpas[37] – is facilitated by gestational stresses. Each genetic strain within a species carries certain potentialities for impairment which will vary from those of another strain. Consequently, in a genetically mixed population, identical prenatal stresses, even at the same stage of pregnancy, may have very varying effects.

In a classic experiment Clarke Fraser and his colleagues[17] demonstrated this genetic-environmental interaction among various strains of mouse. By administering cortisone in mid-pregnancy they obtained the following incidence of cleft palate, according to the particular cross that they bred:

Cross			*% with cleft palate*	*No. of offspring*
mother		*father*		
A	×	A	100	36
C	×	C	17	86
A	×	C	43	46
C	×	A	4	82

From these results the authors concluded that the manifestation of the defect depended upon the genetic constitution both of the foetus and of the mother.

The same seems to apply to man. If the mother has German measles in early pregnancy, there is only about a 20 per cent chance, in a British population, of malformation or serious defect.[38] Similarly, only about one in three of the mentally normal children who constituted the 450 controls of the subnormal sample referred to above[57] had a serious illness during infancy following a disturbed pregnancy. Characteristically, the boy infants were more severely affected (41 per cent) than the girl infants (25 per cent). The risk of congenital malformation or of mental deficiency following a stressful pregnancy is very much less – possibly no more than 1 in 30 or 40. Since only a certain proportion of children are affected in any one way following gestational stress, the impairments are found in loose association rather than tight syndromes. But when the more frequent minor impairments, including disposition to behaviour disturbance, subnormal mental functioning, and poor motor coordination, are taken into account, they occur together sufficiently often to produce the phenomenon of multiple impairment. And this finding may be taken as a fairly good indication of the congenitality of the conditions in question in the individual case.

Implications of Congenital Impairment for Deprivation Studies

The tendency to multiple impairment has important implications for the controversial issue of the effects of early deprivation. During the past generation we have been inclined to account for individual personality differences almost exclusively in postnatal terms, notably in the quality of the early mothering. Where no gross deprivation could be found, it has been suggested that variations in the warmth of maternal affection, in the way the mother held and tended her baby, and so forth, could have disproportionately large effects upon the subsequent personality development of the child. The remarkable thing is the paucity of research results confirming such long-term consequences of deprivation. This is the conclusion reached by three of the four reviewers of the literature in recent years (O'Connor,[44] Yarrow,[81] and Casler[8]). Only the fourth, Ainsworth,[3] insists that deprivation experience may in some cases lead to grave effects that resist reversal. And even she has to rely upon the findings of a single worker, Goldfarb,[21, 22] as 'the chief evidence for the claim that very severe and prolonged deprivation beginning in the first year of life may leave grave, permanent effects on the personality'. Neither Ainsworth nor Goldfarb, however, took the tendency to multiple congenital impairment into account. The basic design of Goldfarb's experiments consisted in comparing institutionalized children who had been placed in adoptive or foster homes at a comparatively early age – soon after birth or within fourteen months – with other children who had been retained in the institution until they were three years old. He found that those placed early, and so less exposed to institutionalization, were more advanced mentally and showed less behaviour disturbance. Goldfarb's work was in general carefully executed and his results were striking. But he did not say why the children in the second group had been retained in the institution whereas the others had been adopted early. One knows that agencies are reluctant to pass for adoption any child who is obviously poorly and ailing, is suspected of being mentally defective, or whose behaviour is giving cause for concern. For such children the prognosis as regards mental ability and social adjustment – as shown by Drillien's work and the Bristol hospital results quoted above – would be relatively poor. The manner in which Goldfarb chose his groups would accordingly have biased his results against institutional care. His findings might therefore be quoted to demonstrate the effects of multiple impairment as much as those of deprivation.

The thesis of the catastrophic effects of institutionalization won ready support because of the observed prevalence of mental inferiority and defective personality among institution-reared children. If, as Ainsworth does, we overlook the possibility of a common congenital factor, the causal connection seems obvious. Yet one has only to reflect how infrequently a child comes into care at an early age without there being good reason for assuming a stressful pregnancy – illegitimacy, a disintegrating marriage, cultural demoralization, or serious illness in the mother.

This is not to say that conditions in some institutions will not reinforce the handicap of mind and personality. If a child has an unforthcoming, confidence-lacking temperament he or she needs special stimulation and encouragement in learning. In the Bristol hospital study all the unforthcoming children who came from poor working-class families were backward; the three unforthcoming middle-class children were all average or superior readers. The effects of unstimulating environment added to congenital handicap have already been seen in Drillien's study in regard to general mental development. In an institution there may be no one fondly watching the child's school progress and providing help where necessary; in order to gain a wide experience of life the child would need to be exceptionally alert and enterprising, with the emotional stability to ponder over and benefit from his experience. These abilities are the opposite of the characteristics – unforthcomingness and restless distractibility – most associated with neural impairment, and most frequently found among institution children.

A few of the more recent deprivation studies provide us with further object lessons in ignoring the tendency to multiple impairment. Bowlby, Ainsworth, and their co-workers[6] chose for a critical test of the effects of early separation a group of children who had been in a sanatorium on account of pulmonary tuberculosis. The hypothesis of multiple congenital impairment would, however, predict that a group of tubercular children would show a greater incidence of behaviour disturbance. It could also have been predicted that the most frequent types of personality defect among them would be unforthcomingness and distractibility, or, as the above authors found, 'day-dreaming (withdrawal of attention), diffidence and lack of initiative and concentration'. A further characteristic of these children was their tendency to get unduly rough during playtime. This, with the lack of concentration, could be part of the inconsequential syndrome. The tubercular children, contrary to the expectation of the authors of this study, showed no tendency to 'affectionless character'. The results support an explanation in terms of multiple congenital impairment rather than of affectional withdrawal resulting from early separation. Indeed, all aetiological studies of earlier deprivation which ignore this possibility must be regarded as inconclusive.

The Biological Rationale of Multiple Impairment

When a phenomenon such as that of multiple impairment is observed we have a right to ask, before accepting the explanation that it is congenital in origin, with some kind of genetic basis, how it could have survived the process of evolution. Following his finding of a close relationship between stressful pregnancy and impairment in the infant,[57] the present writer had to ask himself a very similar question: How could it be that, against evolutionary probability, the foetus is so vulnerable to outside influences? He put forward the following tentative explanation:[58]

> 'By the crude theory of the survival of the fittest, proneness to malformation and to ill health should have been eliminated during the rough and tumble of the millennia of savagery. The above psychological traumata would notably have been of much more frequent occurrence among primitive man than in our present-day civilization, despite the hardships and hazards of war; and it goes without saying that the presence of a malformation or of congenital weakness of health would be detrimental to the survival of the individual concerned. Students of the behaviour of the social animals, among which man is included, have however noted responses which are undoubtedly detrimental to the individual's

survival but which contribute to the survival of the group. All that behaviour termed "courageous" belongs to this class. We may therefore ask whether the persistence of malformation and juvenile ill health may be explained by their having survival value for the *group*. Just as the occasional male may have to be sacrificed in battle in defence of the herd, may there not be circumstances which demand sterility, miscarriage, or the sacrifice of the infant? To put the question more succinctly, is the continuum of reproductive wastage* phylogenetically a mechanism of fertility regulation? That some mechanism must exist among food-gathering peoples has often been borne in upon anthropologists. To assume that the population is regulated by sheer starvation does not fit the facts, for there is little evidence of chronic undernourishment in such communities, the individual savage being a well-developed specimen capable of leading a strenuous life. If this argument is valid, there would be great survival value to the group in some form of fertility regulation which by and large adapted the size of the herd or tribe to the means of existence without reducing the functioning efficiency of its members by malnutrition. This might be achieved if the reproductive rate itself were in some way responsive to the contemporary food situation. Actual malnutrition during the pregnancy would thus be expected to lead to sterility and infant loss, but such could only occur when the dangerous state of a general semi-starvation was already upon the tribe. Consequently some much finer barometer of shortage would be needed than the fact of starvation itself. Increasing difficulty in finding food would entail foraging further afield, the hardship of treks, clashes with other tribes involving death and injury of some of the menfolk, retaliatory raids during which children might be killed or maimed, unforeseen natural dangers, the terror of strange places, possibly quarrelling and a straining of personal relationships within the tribe. To the risk of general food shortage must be added the particular difficulties of a family deprived of the adult male hunter by illness, injury, or death, which would make an additional child a burden. These calamities constitute just those types of harassment, distress, and shock which were noted in the above study. On biological grounds, therefore, it is feasible that psychological stresses of this character could be an agent limiting fertility.

This supposition is borne out by two further observations which

* The postulate of Warkany and of Pasamanick and his group of a gradation of impairments according to the severity of the prenatal stress.

have previously been accepted as natural phenomena requiring no specific explanation. If, as would appear, the greater part of non-epidemic ill health in the early years is "facilitated" by pregnancy stress, the higher disease and death rate among male infants lends itself to the explanation that the recovery rate of a tribe would be less prejudiced if it was mainly the male infants who were sacrificed in times of temporary hardship. There is also a greater incidence of other types of impairment among males. The second piece of corroboratory evidence is the surprising tendency of weakly infants, with devoted care, to "grow out" their ailments and to become sturdy adolescents – hence no doubt the folk belief that a child's constitution changes at the seventh and fourteenth years. When it is considered that juvenile ill health is at the very edge of the continuum of reproductive casualty, and presumably reflects the milder pregnancy stresses, we can see this constitutional resilience as a mean of countermanding the "death sentence" upon an infant born in hard times, provided conditions improve to the extent of allowing the mother to nurse the child through the delicate early phase. If, on the other hand, the mother is so preoccupied or exhausted as to be forced to deprive it of the special care needed, then it is likely to become a "casualty" or to develop personality characteristics which have the effect of estranging it from the group. . . .

The above theory of fertility regulation would apply in a general way to mental impairment following unfavourable pregnancy conditions in that mental handicap and slowness of reaction would increase the risk of misadventure in a primitive community. All such linkage of the present tentative findings to general principles of ecological interaction must at this stage remain speculative. There remains however the intriguing query as to the extent to which mental development even within the normal range is conditioned by foetal development. It is probably true of all animals, who feed upon other living matter – as opposed to plants, which obtain their food chiefly by chemical conversion of inorganic materials – that any species which becomes too efficient destroys its own food supply, and so destroys itself. If primitive man, as an animal with a highly developed brain as his speciality, became too efficient, this would apply to him also. Any process that tended to lower the mental capacity of a significant number of individuals in times of food shortage would therefore achieve the paradoxical effect of improving the group's chances of survival.'

Invited by Ashley Montagu to develop this theory further, the writer found corroboration of it in numerous field studies of cyclic fluctuations and phases of non-breeding in animal populations, and a certain amount of further evidence of its working in man.[69] In the same year that the latter article was published, there appeared an authoritative study by Wynne-Edwards[80] of mechanisms for the regulation of population numbers in animals. It can consequently be said that a plausible biological-evolutionary explanation of the tendency to multiple congenital impairment is at hand.

It should, however, be emphasized that although the physiological-instinctive mechanisms for restricting population seem to exist in man, they have been supplemented by cultural provisions. Consequently there is not so great a reliance upon the former, and the appearance of impairment in the child following a disturbed pregnancy is a tendency rather than a certainty.

The Medical Quandary

The paradoxical result is that, so long as the crucial importance of the prenatal phase for the future development of the child remains unrecognized, we shall have to reconcile ourselves to having an increasing number of disturbed children and therefore also of potential delinquents. As has been seen, when a child is unhealthy, he is somewhat more likely to come in the vulnerable category as regards behaviour disturbance. Efficient medical intervention to save weakly infants tends therefore to result in an increase in the proportion of problem children. Dr T. Asuni, a medical superintendent in Western Nigeria, has recently observed this happening in that country:[4]

> 'Another by-product of effective Western public health service is the survival of babies whose viability was very much in the balance in the uninfluenced environment. Unfortunately some of these babies turn out to be mental defectives. In the past, these children would not have survived for long, and they did not create any problems. Their survival will create social and educational problems in the near future.'

In Britain and other technically advanced countries improved medical treatment ensures the survival of large numbers of congenitally impaired children, among whom there will always be a proportion whose neural impairment will render them prone to behaviour disturbance. The use of antibiotics in the treatment of respiratory disease is especially apt to produce this anomalous result, since of all the infantile illnesses pneumonia seems most closely related to future mental and emotional handicaps.[61]

A further result of the intervention of medical science is that of enlarging the hard core of severely disturbed delinquents in Britain. Official optimism which led to the closing of some approved schools in the early 1950s has had to be replaced by pleas to establish new ones to meet the increased number of committals. This situation has occurred despite the reluctance of magistrates (often unjustified) to send boys to approved schools and the unrealistic provision of short-term detention centres. Moreover, according to an official report,[12] it has been the experience of many heads of approved schools that they are receiving boys 'who are more disturbed and less responsive to remedial influence than even the more difficult boys received before the war'. One of the consequences has been the falling success rate of boys after licence from approved schools. The proportion not found guilty of further offences during the ensuing three years fell, for senior boys, from 72 to 44 per cent; for those aged thirteen to fifteen, from 67 to 45 per cent; and for those under thirteen, from 59 to 39 per cent.

Progress in physical medicine, in short, has created problems of behaviour disturbance for which we have not been prepared. We cannot, of course, try to put the clock back by reverting to infanticide or by withholding medical treatment from young children as a form of 'weeding out' the possibly disturbed. The problem must be recognized and the care of the emotionally handicapped child brought up to the level of that of the physically handicapped. At present he is seldom diagnosed as such, often being treated peremptorily as a delinquent.

CHAPTER NINE

Types of Maladjustment

The central problem in the study of maladjustment is the classification and description of its various types. Clinically we are able to recognize the recurrence of regular patterns of symptoms, which justifies our describing disturbed children as hostile, withdrawn, depressed, hyperactive, and so on. But the concepts to which such terms refer have grown up impressionistically, and the terms themselves are used loosely and in rather different ways by clinicians according to their different theoretical backgrounds. To give our concepts a valid empirical foundation we have to go back to the observation of actual maladjusted behaviour in many children, and then arrange the symptoms into what would give the cleanest classification. The attempt of the present writer to do this has been reported elsewhere;[75] it resulted in an instrument for diagnosing type and degree of maladjustment as observed in the school, the family, and the institution.[76] The procedure adopted was the trial of successive groupings of the symptoms of disturbed behaviour until it was felt that reasonably stable 'syndromes' had been achieved.

The classification that most readily suggested itself as a starting-point was a division into inhibited, or too little, and demonstrative, or too much, behaviour, such as was conceptually fixed for us by Jung[31] with his terms introversion and extraversion. But, as Jung also found, it soon proved necessary to subdivide these two categories. More detailed study suggested, indeed, that they each comprised a number of distinct reaction patterns, and that the dichotomy of introversion/extraversion was of limited diagnostic value.

Under-reactive Behaviour

Depression

At an early stage of this attempt at classification, inhibited behaviour was divided phenomenologically into 'withdrawal from voluntary contact with adults and other children', and 'lethargy and lack of interest'. The latter was subsequently renamed *depression.* In its milder forms it was seen as variability in response level from day to day, and lack of physical energy; in its somewhat more severe stage there was a tendency, along with more persistent lethargy, to react to disturbance or frustration by irritability and temper; in its most acute stages the child was described as always dejected, apathetic, and lifeless, and as frequently wandering off alone. Essentially, depression consists in a refusal to meet the challenges of life: the affected child temporarily inhibits his normal striving for personal effectiveness and in the more extreme stage renounces sociability because this always involves an element of 'keeping one's end up'. The irritability and flare-ups occur when the child meets frustration, despite his efforts to opt out, or is subjected to other stressful situations.

Withdrawal

Other inhibited behaviour was at first grouped under the heading of *withdrawal.* At the time the writer was strongly under the influence of the fashionable concept of the 'affectionless character', with its implication that all withdrawal is the result of earlier affectional deprivation. The effect of the secure possession of a concept is that observations that cannot be fitted into it tend to be ignored. Nevertheless, the method of studying 'bits of behaviour' and attempting to group them eventually made it clear that non-depressive inhibited behaviour included much more than genuine affectional negativism or withdrawal. The term withdrawal was retained for that which seemed to consist in a rejection of social contacts. But even this concept was insufficiently refined: such a rejection could result either from a defence against affection and friendship, or from a lack of any desire for human relationships. The theoretical distinction should be between, on the one hand, a conditioning against establishing human contacts as a result of having previously failed to make any or being repeatedly let down; and, on the other hand, the absence of or defect in a need for human contacts.

The latter condition is now generally known as autism. Since we are dealing with different ways of not behaving, the signs that distinguish one from another are necessarily subtle, and it is probably impracticable to attempt to distinguish clearly between defensive withdrawal and autism from reports of behaviour, however carefully defined, made by untrained observers. Autism is frequently associated with mental defect or other symptoms of brain damage, and autistic children are sometimes found in stable and affectionate families where gross deprivation would have been out of the question. The impatience with endearments and disregard for personal relationships seen in the withdrawn child may consequently be the result of damage to the neural structures whose function is to ensure social attachment.

The 'independent' child

A cognate group of symptoms was recognized, consisting of a lack of a desire to please adults, with a certain *independence* or indifference about adult attachments. In the groupings of the Bristol Guides it was treated as the milder form of the K syndrome which is discussed below. It might represent a minimal form of autism which hardly exceeds the normal. Its signs as seen in school are that the child, while not shy or withdrawn, is unconcerned about securing any response or notice from the teacher, does not bother to answer questions in class or to work unless watched or compelled, and never comes for help willingly or volunteers to do a classroom job. In the statistical validation of the Bristol Guides syndromes carried out by Giles,[19] the K syndrome was the only one in which the syndromes did not hang together; notably its milder section (items 1 to 9) differentiated themselves as a separate sub-syndrome from the more severe K items.

Unforthcomingness (effectiveness deficit)

Among the delinquents who were the writer's earliest systematic subject of study, inhibited behaviour had to a great extent been genuine withdrawal, in the sense of a defensive self-isolation arising from long experience of affectional deprivation. When large samples of children in ordinary schools were studied it became apparent that there was a class of inhibited or 'introverted' children who were neither depressed nor in any sense defensive or unconcerned about affection. On the contrary, once their unresponsiveness had been overcome, they were particularly affectionate, helpful, and likeable. Their defensiveness was rather against anybody or anything strange, not against affection in general; in the face of any difficulty they lacked confidence to the extent that they – as their teachers put it – 'retreated into their shell'. Their general manner might be described as 'mousy', and they were unassertive in their relations with other children. This syndrome of *unforthcomingness*, as it was named, seems to consist in an impairment of natural assertiveness or 'go'. In the theoretical frame of reference proposed in Chapter Ten, there is a failure of the process of appraisal in terms of personal effectiveness. A child of this sort would just not feel the challenge to overcome his natural caution in the presence of strangers, to master difficulties, or to 'keep his end up' with his age-mates as regards school attainment, games skills, or venturing farther afield in its neighbourhood.* Needless to say, such children are seldom a nuisance or spiteful to others, and when only mildly affected pass as 'quiet types'. Once again, they are found in stable affectionate homes as well as in depriving situations. Among a group of 142 backward children studied by intensive case-study methods, unforthcomingness was the predominant form of behaviour disturbance (42 per cent of the cases compared with 36 per cent with all other types of behaviour disturbance).

One's first impression may be that this unforthcomingness in backward children is a simple reaction to failure. Undoubtedly it is accentuated thereby, and the affected child tends to brighten up when the teaching method employed enables him to succeed at a task. But the lack of confidence seems a pervasive approach to life, whereas the normally confident child can abandon a task found too hard and turn to another without losing confidence. Furthermore, the unforthcoming child is content not to achieve a greater effectiveness or mastery, and wants only not to be pressed to do so. If this temperamental handicap is due to some defect in the motivational structure we have to consider that it and the mental retardation may have a common origin. In the general study of the causes of mental retardation discussed in the previous chapter, unforthcomingness emerged as one of a syndrome of multiple impairment related to stressful pregnancy.[57, 59] Moreover, the stresses related to unforthcomingness were mainly those occurring in the later stages of the pregnancy, as opposed to those associated with malformation in the child, which were in the early stages. There is thus good reason to believe that

* The characteristics of unforthcomingness as above described apparently formed an important part of Jung's concept of the introvert. Of the latter he writes:[31] 'Strange new objects excite fear and distrust, as though concealing unknown dangers; objects long rooted and blessed by tradition are attached to his soul as by invisible threads; every change has a disturbing, if not actually dangerous aspect.'

unforthcomingness is the outcome of a kind of congenital damage analogous to that causing autism, with the difference that in unforthcomingness it is the neural structure responsible for ensuring personal effectiveness that is impaired, whereas in autism it is that concerned with social attachments.

The K syndrome

In the more serious K type of maladjustment, unconcern about adult attachments or approval was seen to reach the point where it gives rise to antisocial behaviour. From a very early age a normal child learns what causes annoyance to adults, what they disapprove of, and what is likely to provoke a breach of good relationships. His sensitivity to such things rests upon his paramount need for adult attachments and for approval. His knowledge of specific rights and wrongs, although acquired by experience (including, of course, verbal communication), thus has a foundation in instinct. If the latter is absent there is nothing to appeal to, and the child seems to have no 'moral sense'; he feels no guilt at wrongdoing, wants no forgiveness, seeks no sympathy, and has little compunction about doing harm to other people. In his quest for personal effectiveness he is not limited to those opportunities that are socially acceptable; he can exercise dominance by bullying or being spiteful to other children, is likely to be dishonest at games, will take advantage of a position of trust, and may steal so cunningly that he is hard to catch. Likewise he is a clever liar, because he has no guilt to give him away. Children of this kind may appear deceptively normal, since they are not subject to the frustration of being in an unfavourable human situation and so show little emotion or distress. But they are soon found out by their age-mates as having no 'sense of decency' or of comradeliness, and they do not keep a friend long.

Caution is needed in generalizing about the origin of such psychopathic conditions. It is quite usual to find a boy who has completely 'written off' the adult world and adult values, yet shows considerable anxiety for the approval of his age-mates (the XC syndrome). This suggests that the unconcern for adult attachments is the result of earlier deprivation or affectional discontinuity (abandonment by a favourite adult figure). Among delinquent youths one sees instances of this type of 'affectionless character' in relation to gross deprivation.[55] On the other hand, the attitude to age-mates may be more a matter of seeking approval and admiration – by showing off and feats of daring – than a genuine desire for group acceptance. If it were the latter, one would expect a greater care about losing friends. Such juvenile 'psychopaths' are sometimes found in families in which it is hard to imagine gross deprivation, so that for this syndrome also we have to consider the possibility of neural impairment.

In sum, the various types of inhibited or 'introverted' behaviour – withdrawal, autism or quasi-autism, depression, and unforthcomingness – have only a superficial and external resemblance to each other in that they are characterized by a diminution in the amount of activity. Some seem to be caused more by congenital damage than by emotionally depriving experiences. Of those, such as defensive withdrawal and depression, which are more likely to result from deprivation or other stress, we do not know what differences of stress tolerance may induce different reactions or differing degrees thereof in particular children. There is at any rate no simple relationship between these types of behaviour disturbance and postnatal influences.

Over-reactive Behaviour

When exposed to empirical treatment the other side of the traditional dichotomy – that of extraverted or demonstrative behaviour – has also to be broken up into modes of reaction that have little in common except that they are excessive in relation to the situation. Each seems to be based upon different executive mechanisms and to some extent upon different instinctive needs.

Normal attachment behaviour

For the child one of the paramount needs is that of attachment to the guardian adult. Schaffer and Emerson[51] have demonstrated that from the age of seven months there begin to appear behavioural modes which normally ensure attachment to a particular parent figure – smiling, appreciation of cuddling, distress at losing contact, fear of strangers, following, and so on. Each appears spontaneously in the process of maturation, but in no absolutely fixed sequence and at rather variable ages. In the present writer's opinion Schaffer and Emerson's careful empirical analysis provides strong evidence that each of these modes can be regarded as a distinct executive mechanism which has had survival value as a good means of ensuring attachment at the particular phase of development. In some otherwise normal children one or other may be abnormally late in appearing, or fail to appear. Thus some children, from infancy on, are impatient of cuddling but like to be near the guardian adult; others may like cuddling but are unconcerned about keeping within hailing distance (in extreme cases being chronic wanderers). There is also great variation in the degree of anxiety shown following a phase of separation.[50]

Once the child becomes fully mobile he is able to explore further afield, to practise diverse skills, and to exploit a wide range of opportunities for development and personal effectiveness. At this stage the need for attachment takes more 'psychological' forms. The normally secure child does not have to be continually within sight or hearing of the adult, but needs to know that he can make his way back to the home base when he wants to. He learns to value the *quality* of the relationship with the adult. If he acts in a way that makes the adult angry he recognizes the situation as a dangerous one, which if allowed to continue could lead to rejection. Consequently, when he has been 'naughty' and has evoked a disapproving reaction in the adult, he seeks forgiveness. He does this in the form of behaviour – offering to help, coming for love, possibly crying as a means of inducing sympathy – calculated to get himself in the adult's 'good books' again. In normal children one also observes a strong general need for approval: the child brings drawings or objects that he has made or found, and he appreciates symbols of acceptance such as holding hands when out walking.

Attention-seeking

When these executive mechanisms ensuring attachment are resorted to over-readily we speak of *attention-* and *affection-seeking*. In the classroom the normally active child is willing or keen to help the teacher with a job, but some are over-keen, and pester the teacher. These latter will be over-eager to greet, and make excuses for contact with the teacher which might win them appreciation or approval, such as bringing trivial objects found lying in the classroom, constantly offering small gifts or flowers that they have picked, showing drawings and objects they have made, or bringing up their work unnecessarily. In the more extreme cases the child may tell tales about other children's misdoings in order to curry favour, yarn to the teacher – sometimes in a fantastic manner – about his own or his parents' exploits or possessions; he may come with minor bumps and scratches or, failing these, pretend that he has been hurt by another child.

There can be no doubt that often such affection- and attention-seeking derive from anxiety about the maintenance of secure attachments. In many cases the child is patently seeking substitute attachments to compensate for the insecurity of his own family setting. The quest for surrogate parents may induce the child to help the milkman or other tradesmen on their rounds, or a shopkeeper in his shop. He may attach himself to a gang of roadmen or to an allotment-gardener. Sometimes the affection-hungry child will take up with an individual on the lookout for a victim for sexual malpractices.

Nevertheless, caution must again be exercised in concluding that parental failure is always at the root of affection- and attention-seeking. There are great differences between individuals of all ages in their degree of anxiety proneness. Where, as is often the case, phases of affection anxiety (as we may call this behavioural mode) alternate with phases of hostility, we shall be on surer ground in inferring that the child is being deprived of security in his own family. Where a rejecting hostility is in conflict with an intense need for attachments the attention-seeking may take the form of bad behaviour, which demands the teacher's attention even at the risk of punishment. Such a child may also want to monopolize the teacher's affection, resent attention to other children, over-exploit any sign of interest and sulk if an attempt is made to restrain his inordinate demands. On the other hand, instances of attention-seeking are found without the least trace of hostility. In the course of the item validation of the Bristol Guides, behaviour of this sort, which would be regarded as indicating disturbance in older children, was frequently observed among other normal five- to seven-year-olds. Children of this age are evidently less restrained in their attachment demands.

The growing child is progressively conditioned to restrain his instinctive attachment mechanisms. The constant demanding of attention when the adult is busy or tired becomes a nuisance, and is rebuffed by rebuke or irritability. The child's consciousness of no longer being a baby makes him spontaneously restrain his inclination to be cuddled, to be dependent upon the adult for continual approval, or to come for sympathy when hurt. Even though 'spoiled' at home – that is to say, never having been taught to respect the social conventions or the rights of adults – a normal child will rapidly adapt himself to the discipline of a school or of his peer-group. On the other hand, a child who has suffered neural impairment may be relatively unconditionable or without this consciousness of his status as a not-baby. A case that caused the writer much thought some years ago was that of a boy of eight years in a special school who, quite evidently, had a secure and affectionate – possibly too affectionate – family. His three elder siblings were stable and in regular jobs, which may be regarded as confirming the normality of the family setting. Yet this boy had been excluded for a year from school as unmanageable. His tempers were described as appalling; any frustration would occasion an all-out rage during which he would throw milk bottles or hurt other children. But his greatest nuisance was his uncontrollable attention- and affection-seeking. He would be constantly bursting into the headmistress's room or engage any adult who would tolerate him. To multiply opportunities for contact he would think of dodges such as coming three times for three separate pennyworths of biscuits. The headmistress said she had never known a child more in need of affection. Similarly with his mother, on leaving for school he would come back two or three times for an extra hug and to say goodbye again. His attention- and affection-seeking seemed merely to be the operation, in their unconditioned state, of the executive mechanisms ensuring attachment in a young child. The neural structures which would normally be the seat of conditioning or of control had evidently suffered damage. There can be no reasonable doubt that he had suffered brain damage from anoxia at birth. The umbilical cord was wound several times round his neck, and he was 'blue' for over a week. As a baby he was unduly placid, but began to exhibit the terrific tempers from toddlerhood. Up to seven years his vocalizing consisted only of noises, and at eight years he was difficult to understand since he could not pronounce different consonants in succession. He had very poor limb coordination and was slightly athetoid, with constant twitches and jerks. The lesson of this case is that indiscriminate attention-demanding can be an effect of brain damage. Naturally, such a diagnosis would need to be corroborated by other indications and, if possible, by the history.

Aggression

The interpretation of demonstrative behaviour of a hostile or aggressive type suffers from the confused use of these terms. *Aggression* means such different things to people with differing interpretative systems and has so invaded the popular jargon as to have lost its value as a description of a behavioural mode. In the early stage of the work on the Bristol Guides, when members of staffs of children's homes were asked to describe individual children, they would repeatedly say of a child that 'He is very aggressive'. The actual behaviour to which they referred was found, according to the individual, to be assertiveness or dominance (always wanting to be leader or to have his own way), depressive irritability (snapping back at people), hostility or resentfulness, teasing or spiteful molestation, or quarrelsomeness. It is true that all these sorts of behaviour are associated with a degree of physical violence against another person, but basically they have just as little in common as the various types of inhibited or introverted behaviour.

There seems to be a very primitive mechanism of attack which, in the more restrained guise of resentment, comes into play in everyday life mainly in relation to threats against personal effectiveness. People resent being involuntarily deprived of private possessions to a greater degree than they resent the actual loss. The victim of a petty theft may remark indignantly, 'I would willingly have given it to him'. Remarks that are belittling or disrespectful are similarly resented, as is also being ignored. We may swear at a piece of work that has gone wrong, or blame the tool, sometimes throwing away or destroying the offending object. When a sentence won't come out right the sheet of paper may be crumpled and thrown impatiently but harmlessly into the basket. How basic and spontaneous is this impulse to destroy or remove the offending object can be seen from the way children resort to it upon the frustration of any intense desire. A child in a children's home was told that he would have to hand over a pop-gun to the housemother. Rather than do so he broke it across his knee, saying that if he could not use it he would rather break it. A student reported that when she was about six years old she was given a doll's house; apparently because she had been naughty her mother threatened to take it from her and give it to someone else, whereupon she smashed it to pieces.

Hostility

Frustration in personal attachments generates the same mechanisms of attack and removal/avoidance. Once it becomes apparent that an affectionate relationship cannot be established even by making special efforts at propitiation, the offending person is converted from a loved one into an enemy. Hence the traditional fury of unrequited love. The *hostility* – which is the most exact term for this behavioural mode – serves as a means of annulling a love relationship. The desire for love is so crucial and intense that it cannot be assuaged merely by turning to another love object; it has first to be destroyed by substituting hate. Such is the normal course of human passion, and it has value in enabling hopeless or unreliable attachments to be broken and new ones made. The wronged lover often marries 'on the rebound'. During the process of affection-killing, however, there may be active spite and a wish to injure. This is followed by a phase of denying that the loved one was ever worthy of love, and every possible fault is found in him or her in the same way as the fox of the fable decided that the unattainable grapes were sour anyway. But this form of compensation can be used only after the love has been killed by a phase of violent hostility.

As a reaction against affectional disappointment or rejection, hostility has much in common, outwardly, with the simpler attack mechanism. One may even suppose it to have evolved therefrom. Just as, in the evolution of the organs of the body, one function overlies another – the nose for breathing and smelling, the tear-ducts for moistening the eyeball and for weeping – so we may expect one executive mechanism to have a certain duality of function or to overlap another. Hostility seems to be an extension of the primitive attack mechanism in that it has the additional function of breaking an unreliable affectional bond.

The child who is deprived of reliable family attachments reacts by hostility against the offending parent. During quarrels with her husband or in phases of depressive irritability the mother may threaten to desert the home, and may make realistic gestures of doing so. In moods of exasperation against the child the father may threaten to disown him or have him put in an institution. When such threats are construed merely as expressions of annoyance their effect is usually to arouse moderate anxiety, which induces the child to mend his ways or to become very helpful in the home in order to make life easier for the mother. But at the stage when the child becomes convinced that his parents are prepared to abandon him the situation becomes intolerable, since reliable adult attachments are a primary need in childhood. From his case studies of delinquents the writer observed that a single loyal parent could meet this need, whether it be the mother or the father. In confirmation of this finding McCord and McCord[42] found that 'rejection by one parent did not produce a significantly higher crime rate than that for boys whose parents were both loving. So long as the mother was loving, crime rates rose only slightly if the father was rejecting. . . . If, on the other hand, the father was loving, the attitude of the mother did not make a significant difference.' A high incidence of crime – 70 per cent compared with 32 to 46 per cent for the other combinations – occurred when both parents were rejecting.

As a type of maladjustment, hostility must be understood as a relationship-severing mechanism. This explains the frequently met anomaly of the boy who, while showing unmistakable signs of affection towards his mother, commits hostile acts against her or behaves in a manner calculated to cause her distress. In such cases one may suspect that the boy looks to his mother as the main source of affection, but that the mother, under the strain of quarrels with her husband or of his antagonism to the boy, lapses into a state of irritable-depressive rejection or supports the father's threats of putting away 'for the sake of the family peace'. Her unreliability induces an intolerable anxiety which can be ended only by a breaking of the love relationship. The summoning up of hostility – the substitution of hate for love – enables the boy to do this. It is a violent counter-emotion, and gives rise to provocative behaviour by which the doer invites rejection and hostility against himself. It is quite different from the rage of the cerebrally impaired child or from the phases of defiance exhibited by the ordinary boy in moments of frustration against restraint. The hostility towards the parents takes the form of sullen, uncooperative, bloody-minded moods, stealing from the parents, usually in a way that does not admit of concealment, or stealing from friends, relatives, or lodgers with the result that the parents become embroiled with them or are brought to shame. The hostile child is likely to cause anxiety by going missing for hours at a time, truanting, or running away from home. After a family crisis or some patent evidence of the loved parent's disloyalty he may rob the gas meter and run away, subsequently committing a series of flagrant delinquencies. Often the hostility is transferred to the adult world in general; the boy seeks the company of similarly antisocial types and indulges in systematic delinquency. In his hostile moods he no longer values his attachment to his family and so he is freed from the fear of evoking disapproval. Since rebuke and punishment are effective only as symbolic threats of the withdrawal of love, they mean nothing to the hostile child except to confirm his feelings of being unloved. This confirmation in turn produces a redoubling of the hostile acts. It is also understandable that behaviour calculated to secure rejection usually has this effect. The exasperated parent may be excused in entering a plea of 'beyond control' and vehemently demanding the removal of the child. Consequently, the vicious circle of rejection threats by the parent and mounting hostility in the child may make temporary removal from the house imperative.

Delinquency with hostile motivation is often accompanied by an unconscious – or even sometimes a conscious – desire for removal. The child may commit offences without the least concealment, and commit further ones of a provocative character while awaiting the court hearing, so that the magistrate sums him up as a potentially wanton criminal who must be dealt with in an exemplary fashion. It will be recalled that on the day of his court appearance Arthur (p. 41 above) stole his parents' belongings and pawned them. As far as the child is concerned, indeed, hostility may be viewed as a self-banishing mechanism.

Because hostility is an affection-killing mechanism it is only in evidence so long as the affection is not yet dead. Beneath it there is always anxiety. From time to time, according to the occasion and the child's capacity to resist stress, the anxiety may reassert itself. This often happens once the child's removal has been effected; then, in a remand home or approved school, he becomes very homesick, tries to run away back home, and acts as if he had never been hostile or sought removal. Hostility is also a very variable and unstable mode of behaviour. If the child can be convinced of the adult's loyalty and reliability as a source of affection, it may collapse and be replaced by anxiety for acceptance. Consequently the hostile child is usually amenable to a form of situational treatment which consists in providing security of this kind and avoiding threats of rejection.

Hostility towards adults outside the family circle is a matter of the transfer of the attitude from the home or other attachment situation. In school, hostility can be recognized by uncooperative moods or a constant sullenness, bad behaviour which can be distinguished from mere indiscipline by its unnecessarily provocative character, aggressive defiance when corrected, and association with other antisocial children. A mere readiness to resort to violence or passing expressions of antagonism are not in themselves evidence of hostility as defined, since they can be the result of brain damage or other failure of the controlling mechanisms.

It follows that when the child in school shows the syndrome of hostility, the causes must be sought in the home or analogous situation. It is hardly likely that, as a characteristic attitude, it will be aroused in a stable child by a teacher. When emotionally stable children dislike the way they are treated by an adult outside the family they react, except under extreme provocation, by being guarded in their responses so as not to give cause for unpleasantness. Naturally, a liked teacher and a happy school atmosphere will evoke cooperative attitudes and tend to allay any readiness to hostility that may exist, and a knowledgeable teacher can play a therapeutic role by refusing to be provoked into taking up the position of an enemy.

Whereas of all the types of maladjustment hostility seems the most directly related to family insecurity, it would be a mistake to regard it as solely the product of defective parent/child relationships. There is also the factor of differing vulnerability to stress. This was well exmplified in a backward boy of nine years, who was the youngest of several stable brothers, most of whom had left school and were regular wage-earners. The mother was an affectionate woman, but subject to moods of depressive irritability during which she threatened to clear out. The boy admitted that this worried him greatly, but when asked what his brothers thought of this possibility he replied quite shortly, 'They say she won't'. In one member of a family who is emotionally robust such threats go unheeded, in another who is temperamentally hypersensitive they generate anxiety. It is possible that there is an element of weakness of temperament in all cases showing marked hostility. Among approved school boys whose delinquency takes the pattern of running away and committing offences following bad relationships with the parents, one often notices a general impulsiveness, high emotional reactivity, high face colour, and quick reversion to immature behaviour. Indeed, as Prechtl[46] points out, the tiresomeness and nuisance of a neurally impaired child from early infancy may have been the reason for his rejection by the mother. Similarly, the father may regard such a child as a black sheep who is better removed from the family before the other children pick up his bad ways. The degree to which behaviour disturbance of a hostile type has its origin in congenital impairment can be judged only on the evidence of collateral neural damage obtained by a careful taking of the history from birth. The phenomenon of multiple impairment which has been discussed in earlier chapters provides a set of criteria for the congenital origin of behavioural abnormality.

Hostility viewed as self-banishment from the family unit requires explanation in terms of survival. As a means of quickly breaking unreciprocated affectional attachments among young adults it has obvious advantages in curtailing destructive rivalries and facilitating reattachment to a third party. In cultures where the unwanted child can similarly break the affectional bond with his own parents and attach himself to another family or another adult within the wider family group, he would presumably have an increased chance of survival. In wild animal populations, however, similar behaviour is virtually suicidal. Rejection of the young and the latter's forced emigration are associated with over-population.[69] The young show other signs of 'maladjustment', notably a loss of the instinctive behaviour ensuring their own safety. In the case of the lemming there is a built-in suicidal urge always to run downhill, so that the emigrants eventually reach the sea and are drowned. The behaviour of the emotionally disturbed hostile child 'on the run', with his indifference to exposure and isolation from human contact except to steal, would be equally suicidal under tribal conditions of life. If a child is left uncherished because of the shortage of food and the social stresses that go with human over-population, it is unlikely that neighbouring families will be any better off. There is thus reason to believe that the self-banishing aspect of hostility in the child has had survival value for local populations in reducing excess numbers, in the same manner as population-regulating mechanisms operate in virtually every species of animal.[80] When the stresses arising from over-population reach a certain level of intensity the normal instinctive patterns of behaviour are replaced by apparently equally instinctive patterns of destructive stress behaviour in the affected (mostly young) animals. Hostility in human beings would seem to be a relic of this self-annihilatory response. It is not simply a matter of behavioural breakdown or disintegration, but of the substitution of a different behavioural mode; the patterning of the syndrome is unmistakable, with the regular appearance of its elements in case after case.

In *Man Meets Dog*, Lorenz[36] recounts an incident which demonstrates that hostility springing from desertion is not confined to the human species. A bitch which he had trained had become very attached to him, and this attachment survived a separation of four months. When, however, she noticed the packing of cases and other signs of his impending second departure she became very depressed and refused to leave his side. It was decided to shut her up when the point of leaving came, but then she kept her distance and all attempts to catch her failed. On the way to the station she followed at a little distance with lowered tail, ruffled mane, and wild eyes. She succeeded in boarding the train while it was moving and had to be thrown off again. During the following weeks she roamed the district, carried out many depredations upon neighbours' hens, lost her house-training, refused to obey anybody, and became increasingly ferocious. This episode has innumerable parallels in the 'running amuck' of delinquent boys prior to their entry to, or as absconders from, approved schools.

A child's behaviour in relation to his age-peers is usually the reflection or counterpart of that which he exhibits towards adults. Hostility towards other children (HC) tends to accompany that towards adults, but mostly remains at the stage of the simpler attack mechanism. Typically, the hostile child will be a member of an antisocial gang that may molest or be otherwise antagonistic to outsiders. Since by temperament children of this type are over-quick reactors, they are likely to get involved in fights, and are easily provoked by teasing. In the more extreme cases their relations with other children are constantly bad and on the verge of actual hostilities. Again, however, it is important to make a distinction where possible between hostility to other children originating in family insecurity and the uncontrolled rage responses of the neurally impaired child. Children of the latter type are sometimes teased or provoked because they can be relied upon to over-react by impotent retaliation.

The easily led, showing-off syndrome

The syndrome of anxiety for the approval and affection of other children (XC) probably represents a mixture of executive mechanisms, and could no doubt be usefully subdivided if a sufficient number of cases were studied. On the one hand there is the element of genuine anxiety for acceptance by other children, such as may induce a boy to steal surreptitiously from members of his own family in order to have the means to buy the favour of a gang leader. Boys of this type may have no personal inclination towards delinquency, but come in the class of what the probation officer describes as *easily led*: they cannot resist the invitation of others to take part in a housebreaking or in the driving away of a car. There can be little doubt that this anxiety for acceptance is an attempt by the insecure boy to find substitute attachments with his age-peers or somewhat older boys. It is significant that it is virtually never found apart from other types of maladjustment, and is notably associated with the set rejection of adult attachment (K syndrome). The family background is usually that of uncertainty or distance as far as the parents are concerned; in many cases the child was reared by surrogate parents or developed a primary attachment to another adult, so that no firm affectional bond was established with the true parents in the early years. Sometimes the true parent has been rejected in favour of (usually) a spoiling grandmother, so that the uncertainty about the mother's affection almost amounts to estrangement. This divided maternal attachment is one of the more common types of family situation conducive to maladjustment, incidences of which have been quoted in Part I.

The other element in the XC syndrome is analogous to the common tendency of children to show off. It may indicate an anxiety for acceptance, in cases where the affected child is unable to resist being 'dared' to commit foolhardy acts, including destructive vandalism. Barring the possibility of cerebral impairment, a child who values his family attachments will hold back from such escapades because of the parental disapproval that would be incurred; consequently there may be some underlying defect in the parent/child relations when the child yields to such temptations. French[18] found that boys convicted of vandalism were slightly more maladjusted as a group than the general run of Glasgow boys put on probation.

Nevertheless, showing off is sometimes found in brain-damaged children, and among those who rank as mentally normal the tendency can be present in various degrees. Any child in whom the effectiveness-appraisal system* and its executive mechanisms are in healthy operation is constantly exploring new means of dominance, control, display, etc. When any of these, such as obstreperousness which becomes dangerous or a nuisance, are disapproved of by the adult world, the child is subjected to a process of conditioning against such behaviour. In certain instances a mild degree of cerebal impairment may make the child resistant to this conditioning. Discerning diagnosis must weigh up these alternatives by taking the collateral indications into consideration.

Distractibility

The only type of behaviour disturbance remaining to be considered among those identified by the Bristol Guides is *restlessness* (R) or *distractibility*. As a descriptive category it is undoubtedly valid, since this type of disorganized motivation is not infrequent. As a concept, however, it fails to give satisfaction because it is purely phenomenological. For understanding we want to be able to relate phenomena. The restlessness syndrome occurs frequently along with other patterns of maladjustment, and it is tempting to interpret it as a by-product of anxiety. On the other hand it is, next to unforthcomingness, the commonest type of behaviour disturbance among the mentally subnormal, which suggests neural impairment. Children of this type often possess remarkable powers of observation and perceptual discrimination, but nothing is attended to for more than a fleeting moment. Göllnitz[24] has described the condition as that of being percept-dominated. Neurologically it could be regarded as an

* See Chapter Ten, below.

inability to inhibit afferent stimuli, such as is necessary if we wish to concentrate or ponder upon a given topic. Because of the failure to conceptualize that this entails the child remains at a low level of mental development. Children who are less severely affected will be unable to deal with concepts requiring any degree of abstraction, but may function satisfactorily at the concrete level and give a superficial appearance of brightness and perkiness. The reader will recognize the type in the inconsequential boys described in the case studies.

The inconsequential syndrome

The central feature of *inconsequence* is an inability to operate on a time dimension. The normal human being aims to maintain his social attachments, his status with others, and his personal effectiveness through time. Although he may be subject to immediate stimulus-response impulses in that he *feels* like doing something rash, he usually restrains himself if the actual behaviour is liable to have unwelcome consequences. He does this by substituting for the immediately provoking stimulus situation a visualization of himself as an organism functioning into the future; thus he still obeys the laws of stimulus and response, but with a time dimension. In popular language we say that by restraining his impulse or having regard for the future he exercises an act of will; in psychology Hearnshaw[27] has proposed the term 'temporal integration'.

The advantage of this concept is that it enables us to bring inconsequential and distractible behaviour within the theoretical framework outlined in the next chapter. The failure of temporal integration seems to occur at the stage of appraisal: owing presumably to some impairment of the neural structures that enable us to envisage ourselves as in situations-through-time, the acts of appraisal in terms of favourableness or unfavourableness which generate behaviour are restricted to the immediate situation. The result is naturally a larger number of 'extraverted' responses, many of which will be damaging to the best interests of the doer and his associates.

Failure of temporal integration includes also an inability to take account of the results of previous behaviour. A typical comment by the teacher about a child of this sort is that he is too immature to heed correction, and by the parent that he is irrepressible and never bears resentment. In short, the inconsequential child is resistant to conditioning. This unconditionability seems to have two aspects. First, correction, punishment, approval have little or no effect because attention is distracted by a new stimulus before the record can be formed in the brain.[45] Rats 'punished' by an electric shock when they go to the wrong food dish mostly fail to learn if the distinguishing sign is simultaneously withdrawn, and we often fail to remember the name of the person to whom we are introduced because of our preoccupation with the personal situation. In popular language, the inconsequential child does not give himself time to rue the results of his misconduct. Some of those in the case studies were irrepressible and puckish, and attractive owing to their ability to 'come up again smiling'. The second aspect of this unconditionability is a general impulsiveness, or failure to ponder prior to acting. That is to say, even if learning has taken place in the sense that a record has been made in the brain, it is not utilized. Such children resort to thoughtless guesses and give hit-and-miss answers, although when encouraged to think for a moment they easily see the right one. In their general behaviour, similarly, they know the right thing to do, but obey a thoughtless impulse. They may respond to an invitation from other boys to perform foolish pranks; they figure among the 'easily led' type of delinquent.

In defining a syndrome of inconsequence, however, we come up against a complication. The kind of impulsive behaviour in which the affected child tends to indulge will depend upon what his main needs are. If they are chiefly those of personal effectiveness, he may satisfy them by any sort of hedonistic 'one-up-manship' that opportunity offers. He may show off, clown, play to the gallery, and try to 'take the mickey' out of his teacher. If, on the other hand, his more urgent need is for affection and social attachment, he may appear as an attention-seeker. In the discussion of a brain-damaged boy of this sort earlier in this chapter the suggestion was made that his attention-seeking was not the result of deprivation but just that he had never become conditioned by the rebuffs of the adults whom he importuned. Thus some inconsequential children will play adults up; others will pester them thoughtlessly and tire them with constant chatter.

Whereas the symptoms of inconsequence were observed, as instances of maladjusted behaviour, in the course of the compilation of the Bristol Guides, the syndrome as such had not then been formulated. As a first step to its identification, the items marked for the eight inconsequential cases among the thirty-three troublesome children were tabulated, and seventeen were found to occur three or more times in all of them. Their mean item-frequency per 100 cases was 52·1, whereas the corresponding frequency among the 130 assorted maladjusted boys of the final sample used for item-validation was only 29·2.[75] Among the 110 of the unsettled group it was 20·8, and among the stable only 9·8. Since these results indicated an objective foundation for the syndrome, the truants and their controls were combed through to find further boys with the same characteristics. The criteria used were that they should have at least six indications of behaviour disturbance, and that half or more of their total scores should be composed of the above seventeen items. A *prima facie* validity for the syndrome was established since, in the resulting final sample of nineteen inconsequential boys, thirteen symptoms occurred at least seven times. Provisionally we may take these, as listed in *Table 34*, as the core items for the syndrome. Other near-qualifiers, with the number of times that they occurred given in parentheses, were:

XA 8 Sidles up to or hangs around teacher (5)
XA 3 Over-talkative, tires with constant chatter (5)
D 8 Flies in a temper if provoked (6)

The first two typify the attention-seeking inconsequential child, and in a larger sample would probably qualify for the syndrome. The last is more typical of what is regarded as brain damage.

The two last items in *Table 34*, D 13 and D 1, seem incongruous, but again the explanation may be that inconsequence merges with other behavioural effects of neural dysfunction. Rather than clear-cut syndromes we observe tendencies or jumps on a frequency distribution. The slumping and lolling about of the inconsequential boy recall the lassitude that Göllnitz[24] listed as one of the characteristics of the brain-damaged child. In common with other authorities he mentions lability of mood, which probably accounts for the high frequency of the item 'sometimes eager, sometimes doesn't bother' in answering questions. On the other hand, inconsequential children may slump and loll about because they have resisted the cultural conditioning which induces normal children to bear themselves 'correctly'.

The only girl among the thirty-three troublesome children who exhibited the characteristics of inconsequence was Rose in Group II, but her dominant type of maladjustment was hostility, with a score of 11, so that she could not be used in the identification of a syndrome. Among the children of the validation sample quoted above the preponderance of inconsequence among boys was equally striking. The mean frequency rate of the inconsequential items was twice as high for boys as for girls among the unsettled, and nearly twice as high among the stable. Much of the restlessness and immaturity held to

Table 34 Frequency of 13 inconsequential items among 19 boys who scored heavily on those items

Coding on BSAG	*Item*	*Frequency*
R 5	Careless, untidy; often loses or forgets books, pen	9
R 9	Cannot attend or concentrate for long (cannot sit still when read to or during broadcasts, plays with things under desk, etc.)	12
R 2	Starts off others in scrapping and rough play	8
R 1	Gets very dirty during day	8
R. 10	Does not know what to do with himself, can never stick at anything long	7
R 6	Rough and ready, slapdash (in manual work)	10
R 11	Too restless to remember for long (after correction)	8
XA 10	Constantly needs petty correction	11
XC 11	Misbehaves when teacher is out of room	9
XC 14	Foolish pranks when with a gang	8
XC 15	Follower in mischief	7
D 13	Slumps, lolls about	10
D 1	Sometimes eager, sometimes doesn't bother (answering questions)	9

be characteristic of ordinary boys may thus indicate a minimal degree of this form of disturbance. In Chapter Eight the greater prevalence of impairment among males has been proposed as an indication for congenitality.

CHAPTER TEN

A General Theory of Human Motivation

Explanation presupposes a foundation of what we like to regard as established fact. In everyday life we can work from a large number of practical certainties, such as our experiences of gravity, weight, volume, sharpness and bluntness, heat and cold, and the constant properties of known materials. But we have no such tangible and verifiable experience of what causes behaviour. Through the ages, therefore, man has been led to postulate either, as Plato did, a soul as the motive force, with its various parts initiating different types of behaviour; or, as in the case of the philosophers of the Renaissance, that differences in the behaviour of individuals arise from the admixture of the elements of earth, fire, air, and water in each person's constitution. In more modern times instincts, drives, 'motives', or other sources of psychic energy have been made to serve as the explanatory bedrock. Needless to say, there is no means of verifying the existence of any of these supposed bases of human motivation, nor do the facts of behaviour force us to conclude that they must exist. Man has invented them in his attempt to explain himself.

Appraisal as the Forerunner of Behaviour

Let us, then, try to conceptualize behaviour in the most general, self-evident terms. Its value from an evolutionary point of view is that it enables the organism to change its environment in its favour; or, if this is not possible, to escape from an unfavourable or to seek a more favourable environment. To use the formulation of Nissen,[43] the effect of behaviour is to provide near-optimum relations between the organism and its environment. This implies that any living creature, through its sense organs, is constantly – albeit unconsciously – *appraising* its environment in terms of favourableness or unfavourableness. If the appraisal records 'unfavourable', behaviour normally results. Such appraisal will be made in relation to the satisfaction of a deficiency either at the organic level, as for food, drink, mating, etc., or at the psychological level, as for social attachment or dominance.

Are the appraisal-response systems instinctive?

Whether the motivation of behaviour, as this appraisal-response process is now generally called, is instinctually provided or acquired is a matter of much controversy that would require a treatise to itself. Without presuming, therefore, to settle the issue, the writer will refer to two recent empirical studies of young children, which are in addition suggestive for the understanding of certain temperamental defects.

The first is a study by Schaffer and Emerson[51] of the development of social attachments in young children. It raises the question whether these *originate* as intrinsic requirements or are derived from a general need for stimulation. To put the issue more specifically, is the young infant equipped with innately provided means of appraising its situation in terms of human contact and of initiating behaviour when a deficiency is signalled? The most critical data, therefore, are those to do with the *onset* of attachment behaviour. The first point we can note is that smiling at a human face and crying upon its withdrawal appear at a very early age. Schaffer and Emerson found that eight out of ten of the infants in their series were already showing such responses when observations were commenced during the second month.

The earlier the appearance of a behavioural mode the greater the likelihood of its instinctive origin, and the more the onus of showing otherwise falls on those who lean towards explanations in terms of conditioning. Because Schaffer and Emerson began their study only after, in the main, indiscriminate attachment behaviour had already appeared, they could deal only with factors affecting the onset of attachments to particular individuals. If specific attachment to the mother develops as a conditioned response to the 'organic' gratifications derived from her, one would expect that the more concentrated the gratifications the sooner the conditioning would be effected. But Schaffer and Emerson found that the age of onset of attachment to the mother was unrelated to the amount of time she spent with the child (this in fact varying widely, since some went out to work and some did not). It was similarly unrelated to age of weaning, length of the weaning period, and all the variables studied of toilet-training. Their finding parallels Harlow's,[26] that the preference of young Rhesus monkeys for a cloth as opposed to a wire mother surrogate was not related to the source of feeding; the cloth model was preferred even when food was supplied entirely through the wire mother-model. Moreover, 39 per cent of Schaffer and Emerson's series of infants had, by the age of eighteen months, developed first attachment preferences for adults who were not mainly responsible for their feeding, and 22 per cent of the adults chosen (mostly the fathers) took no part in the child's daily care. The authors conclude: 'It appears that attachments may develop even when the individuals to whom they are formed have in no way been associated with physical satisfactions.'

If the development of attachment behaviour were the result of conditioning one would also expect that its intensity would depend upon the amount of stimulation. Such an assumption underlies attempts to account for later affectional deficiency by postulating deprivation of 'maternal warmth' in infancy. Schaffer and Emerson divided their mothers into two groups according to whether their contacts with their children were personal or impersonal. Under the first they included either direct bodily contact as in handling, kissing, cuddling, etc., or visual-audile contact as in talking, cooing, or smiling. The impersonal type of mother diverted attention away from herself by means of toys, novelties, food, etc. None of these variants showed a significant relationship to the intensity of the child's attachment to the mother; those with 'impersonal' mothers were no less attached than the rest.

In sum, neither the time of onset of attachment behaviour nor its intensity can be feasibly attributed to conditioning. The evidence provided by Schaffer and Emerson's work is all the more convincing in that the authors themselves are unwilling to infer an instinctive basis for attachment behaviour as such. (They postulate its origin in a generalized need for stimulation which becomes narrowed down to a responsiveness to human beings because of the gratifications with which their appearance is associated. But if the need itself had its origin in conditioning one would have thought that its development would also have depended thereon, which their study shows not to be the case.)

When an attachment need already exists, the choice of the person to serve as the source of gratification depends, as would be expected, upon conditioning. The children in Schaffer and Emerson's series preferred those adults whom they found most rewarding in the sense of being more responsive. Strong attachments were sometimes formed to individuals who were available for comparatively short periods, provided they were prepared to interact fairly intensely, whereas the infants tended to turn from unresponsive mothers to other more responsive adults. This is but one example of the universal tendency to the selection of the most favourable classes of situation.

The second study is one by the present writer[66] of the development in a young child of behaviour which was not directly related to organic needs or social attachments. In order to exclude possibly random movements only actions for which there was evidence of motivation were taken account of. Such evidence took the form of concentration of attention, perseverance or unambiguous repetition, expressions of gratification or frustration, and priority over organic need. The observations were classified into five main groups according to the type of relationship between the infant and his environment that resulted from his behaviour. These were (1) recognition or discrimination, (2) completion, (3) control, (4) exploration, (5) producing a spectacular change. It was argued that the above could be viewed as aspects of a general relationship of *effectiveness* which the infant sought to establish between himself and his immediate surroundings. Moreover, the relational changes that were preferred at any one stage of development were those that were novel or at the limit of the child's capacity. Thus the need was for a progressive effectiveness, and observation of the unhampered child for a complete day showed that, during his waking hours, when other needs were satisfied, the efforts to establish such relationships were continuous.

Behaviour meeting the above criteria was observed from the age of seventy-eight days, but observations did not begin from birth and were made in diary form before the induction of the general concept of effectiveness-seeking. If, consequently, a similar study was undertaken, still earlier behaviour might be found to meet the criteria. The forty-eight modes of behaviour observed were analysed in order to test the possibility of their having resulted from conditioning in relation to other needs such as organic gratification or desire for approval. For various reasons conditioning was ruled out for thirty of them. Of the remaining eighteen, eight seemed most likely to result from spontaneous imitation, which – it was argued – can most feasibly be viewed as a form of identification, that is to say, an attempt to copy a mode of effectiveness observed in the more powerful adult. The origin of the remaining ten was open to argument, but to insist that they resulted from conditioning would have left the greater part of the observations unexplained and would have had low epistemological status. The early age at which the behaviour in question appeared, and the impossibility of adducing conditioning or other form of learning as a general explanation, justified the conclusion that the infant's attempts to establish these relationships of effectiveness were instinctive.

The concept of needs

It is easy to fall into the way of speaking of a child's *needs* for attachment or effectiveness. There is no harm in doing so provided we do not allow ourselves to conceptualize needs as explanatory entities, and thereby commit the same error as is involved in the postulation of instincts, drives, and motives. When the term 'need' is used – as it often is – throughout this book it is merely a way of saying that, to judge from the results of regularly preferred behaviour, an organism requires and seeks to establish relationships of certain broad types between itself and the environment. Examples are the ingestion of food and drink, avoidance of harm, seeking warmth and comfort, maintaining contact with fellow-members of the species, and – for man and the higher animals – maintenance of a relationship of personal effectiveness, including, where possible, dominance.

When we come to ask what may lie behind these needs or seekings after classes of relationship, we do not have to infer anything more than an appraisal response system as mentioned above. In other words, no entity is at the source of the motivation except a neural structure. It is a system of stimuli and responses within which the former are appraised in terms of fairly wide criteria of favourableness or otherwise. We have to infer the existence of instinctive means of assessing whether the situation meets the needs of the organism as they are at any time, and of links with the behaviour-instigating neural structures. Such a concept of the 'motivation' of behaviour is – sometimes in different terms such as 'filtering' or 'editing' – widely accepted by neurologists, and indeed the fact of appraisal, to use the term preferred by the present writer as having the least metaphorical overtones, is inescapable.

Temporal integration

For man we have to add a corollary that the appraisal in terms of favourableness is in respect of the individual's situation through time, thus obviating the compulsion to respond to each and every unfavourable contemporary situation or stimulus. Provided we possess this capacity for temporal integration we can substitute a concept of an ongoing relationship which it may be more important to maintain at optimum favourableness than the relationship of the moment. The situation, or 'stimulus', to which the individual responds is thus an envisaged one, wider than that which is perceived at any one point of time. The immediate situation is reduced in size to a fraction of the total stimulus and its power is correspondingly diminished.

The Executive Mechanisms

Lorenz has argued convincingly that the instinctive tendency to use each organ must have evolved concurrently with the evolution of the organ itself. For those organs such as the hands and feet, the larynx, and all the large skeletal muscles this amounts to saying that each species has developed the behavioural propensities appropriate to its bodily structure. The fleet-footed antelope is temperamentally equipped for running away, the predatory lion for attacking other animals. We would seem, therefore, to be on reasonably sure ground in inferring the instinctive provision of standard modes of reaction, or *executive mechanisms,** by which near-optimal relationships with the outside world are maintained or established. If, as we have also to assume, these mechanisms are transmitted genetically, their neural counterparts would need to be relatively uniform, well-developed structures.

Their value has been that the creature in its natural habitat is enabled to react – without previous learning – to certain general types of situation. A threat may emanate from an object which can be appraised as 'weaker than me' or as 'stronger than me'. Provided such classifications have a sufficient generality and demand distinct

* The term 'executive behaviour' used by some ethologists is tautological, since all behaviour is executive. This applies even to so-called expressive behaviour, because this either has the function of communicating an attitude to another member of the species (e.g. threat postures), or is the unthinking urge to exploit to the utmost a fulfilling situation (e.g. jumping for joy, shouting from elation).

types of response, there would be an obvious survival advantage in the evolution of unlearnt appraisal-response mechanisms. Thus if the offending object is seen as 'weaker than me', attack will readjust the situation; if it is 'stronger than me', flight is indicated. For each generation to have to learn such reactions afresh would entail an enormous mortality. Similarly, if the source of frustration is some obstacle, the situation would be judged as one likely to yield to manipulation, in which case an executive mechanism involving increased effort comes into play. If the obstacle or problem is appraised as beyond the organism's power or ingenuity, it is abandoned or avoided. Along with this process of appraisal-response go certain feeling-states, such as anger with attack, fear with flight, elation with success, and dejection with failure. Broadly, they can be classified into pleasant and painful emotions. The first induce us to continue within a satisfying situation, and the second make it difficult to tolerate a dangerous or otherwise unfavourable one. Both have learning value in teaching us which situations to seek and which to avoid.

Anxiety

When, in an unfavourable situation, no executive mechanism can be brought into play, the result is a painful feeling-state termed *anxiety*. Its survival value has evidently been in preventing the organism from remaining in a situation which is, by and large, unfavourable to it or to the species. Once the needling of the disagreeable circumstance exceeds the individual's tolerance limit total escape is attempted. This may be seen either as a removal urge, or as the inhibition or mental avoidance of the distressing situation. As was seen in the case studies in Part I, both forms of escape can provoke irrational or maladjusted behaviour in those whose stress-tolerance is abnormally low. Anxiety is a state of temporary helplessness or cluelessness which disappears as by magic once a course of action, however forlorn, is embarked upon. It must, however, be sharply distinguished from the normal activation of the executive mechanisms, which ensures the maintenance of favourable relationships. We must not, in short, adduce anxiety as an intrinsic motive.

Maladjustment as self-destructive stress behaviour

If no means of escape from an acutely unfavourable situation is possible the individual will either resort to one of the types of irrational, and possibly self-destructive forms of pseudo-escape, or inhibit the appraisal of unfavourableness, that is to say, relapse into apathy or depression. In a sense these 'maladjusted' reactions may be conceived of as executive mechanisms which, although inimical or even destructive so far as the individual is concerned, have had survival value for the species in reducing overcrowding. Those members of the local population are eliminated upon whom the stresses of overcrowding bear hardest.

What we broadly view as behavioural breakdown is rather the activation of patterns of stress behaviour. Since these appear with regularity and in standard forms in overstressed individuals we must again assume that they have a genetic and instinctive basis, and are a normal component of human nature; they are abnormal only relative to the executive mechanisms which operate under conditions of tolerable stress. The latter have had survival value by enabling the individual to adapt himself to and make the best of his circumstances; the value of the stress behaviour patterns – to the population – has been in their self-destructiveness.

Impairment of Behaviour

It has been the theme of this study that the onset of behaviour disturbance is not only a matter of exposure to abnormal stress; in some, and possibly all, cases the individual has been rendered susceptible by an impairment of temperament. One might speak equally well of an impairment of motivation, because both terms refer to the general style of response to situations observed in each individual. Any impairment of temperament or of motivation can thus be viewed as resulting from interference with the processes of stimulus and response outlined above, and by inference from damage or dysfunction of the neural structures by which they are implemented.

Unforthcomingness was defined in the previous chapter as an impairment of natural assertiveness. In terms of the present analysis of motivation, we would postulate dysfunction of the effectiveness appraisal system. The unforthcoming child is content with a very modest level of effectiveness, mostly restricted to helping with simple domestic jobs. He does not feel the challenge to solve problems, to keep abreast of other children in their play or work achievements, or to understand his environment. No child of this sort figured in the thirty-three case studies reported in Part I, because these were of troublesome children.

Prominent among them, however, was another type of temperamental impairment which was described as a defect of attachment need. In other words, those neural structures responsible for registering the maintenance of stable human attachments were in a state of dysfunction. The result was that, lacking as they often did a sense of the elementary social decencies such as not stealing from one's belonging-group, the children concerned behaved in socially unacceptable ways. The only reason why some of them were not more completely rejected and brought to book for their misdeeds was that they were charming rogues: they still had at their command the instinctive sign-releasers which secure face-to-face acceptance.

Third, inconsequence was seen as a defect of temporal integration, which means that the past and the future are blinkered off. In neural terms there is a failure of association. We have to assume that before response to a presented stimulus is permitted it has to be 'cleared' by reference to a system which assesses its consequences for the future wellbeing of the individual. If need be the response is inhibited by means of an envisaged widening of the situation as earlier described.

Failure to inhibit response to petty frustration is a well-known feature of brain damage. The writer knew a post-encephalitic youth who would throw his carpentry tool wildly across the room if he made a slip in his work; another youth attacked his teaser with a pitchfork. At a milder level similar reactions are typical of what are described as tempers, and they occur most often when the individual is overstressed. Among many maladjusted children failure of the mechanisms of inhibition produce a general picture of over-reaction and over-emotionality. Possibly this is an aspect of what has been described as a low threshold of stress tolerance. There would nevertheless appear to be some further element in the latter, possibly connected with the neural structures through which the executive mechanisms operate.

The writer has been reluctant to infer that the impairments of motivation described above are always the result of brain damage. Göllnitz[23] has indeed demonstrated cerebral abnormalities in such children by the technique of the pneumencephalogram, and similar types of behaviour disturbance have been observed in individuals who have suffered undoubted tissue destruction. This does not justify us, however, in assuming that such damage has taken place in all cases. All we can reasonably infer is neural dysfunction. In Chapter Five it was suggested that neural dysfunction could be a disturbance of the normal sequence of maturation. We do not yet know how the stages of psychological growth are regulated. But it is evident that alongside the hormonal changes of puberty different social attitudes develop: there is a loss of the extraverted spontaneity of childhood, and the beginning of a sensitivity, which often appears to adults as a hypersensitivity, about 'doing the right thing'. In other words, there emerges a new dimension of appraisal in terms of the individual's standing with his peer-group. It was also pointed out earlier that normal young children are 'inconsequential'. The persistence of this behaviour pattern into a later stage of childhood could be due to a defect of hormonal development.

Alternatively, the neural dysfunction could arise from abnormality of metabolism which impinges on the brain tissue. The nerve cells may be ill nourished, ill supplied with oxygen, or exposed to toxic influences. There are indeed reasons for believing that in many cases the dysfunction may be due to the medium within which the neurones function rather than to actual damage to tissue. The first of these is the variability of the behaviour of many presumed brain-damaged children, from virtual normality one day to unmanageability or extreme lethargy the next. This variability is seen also in some forms of epilepsy, squint, chorea,[47] and motor incapacity (hysteria). A metabolic change resulting from stress could account for it; but so also could a lowered stress-tolerance due to tissue damage. Second, there is the tendency towards recovery from certain types of behaviour disturbance at certain stages of childhood. Hyperkinesis tends to diminish rapidly from the age of 8½–9 years, and may disappear altogether after puberty.[5] The same has also been noted by the present writer with regard to unforthcomingness in boys. It is true that in cases of known tissue damage new links may be formed in time and the function restored. But the aetiologically suggestive feature of recovery from impairment of temperament, of motor control, and of health is that it is so often related to a particular stage of development, to wit that of adolescence. Third, although similar symptoms are observed in cases where there are good grounds for a diagnosis of brain damage, there is no direct evidence of such in a surprisingly large number of cases of neural dysfunction. Of the fifty choreiform-syndrome cases studied by Prechtl and Stemmer,[47] 12 per cent had frequent epileptic attacks and a similar proportion showed epileptic discharges on the EEG records. But in forty-three cases (86 per cent) the EEGs were normal except for short muscle artifacts which corresponded to the choroid twitches. It is probable that any group of children showing neural dysfunction will include a proportion in which this is due to tissue damage, and others in which the condition is secondary to intoxication, malnutrition, or hypoxia of the central nervous system. There may well also be a large mixed group in which tissue damage has reduced the number of neurones capable of a given function, so that, with a smaller safety margin, there is a lowered tolerance of noxious influences. In these cases the position would be analogous to the punch-drunk syndrome, in which functional impairment manifests itself only after cumulative traumata.[77] The present writer came to the same conclusion after study of a sample of mentally defective children who had been subjected to very adverse upbringing: in all there was a history of congenital trauma.[71]

Göllnitz[25] proposes a syndromic axis (*Achsensyndrom*) as the outcome of previous brain damage. The milder end includes overreactivity; distractibility; stimulus domination; variability of mood, of motivation, and of bodily function; and general behaviour disturbance. The more severe end includes symptoms which he considers to be in the main irreversible, and it is these that he attributes more confidently to tissue damage. It comprises emotional explosiveness, rage responses, passivity, loss of insight, slowing-up of the thought processes, and general personality disintegration. The twenty-five cases of overactive behaviour described by Ingram,[29] of whom the majority had epilepsy and other symptoms indicating cortical lesion, seemed more characteristic of the more severe end of Göllnitz's axis. The milder end was typical of many of the over-reacting and inconsequential children of the present study.

A further complication is that both among young animals and among humans – notably identical and other twins – there seems to to be a congenital variation on a dominance-submission dimension. Drawing attention to this, Wynne-Edwards[80] points to its biological utility in establishing a survival order in times of overpopulation. This personality dichotomy was evident in the lion cubs studied by Adamson.[1] It corresponds to the production of unforthcomingness following prenatal stress reported by the present writer[59] in children and by Thompson[78] and Ader and Belfer[2] in rats. If this variation is attributed to brain damage in the literal sense it raises the question of what proportion of any human or animal population is cerebrally intact.

Kennedy and Ramirez (see Birch[5]) sum up the present state of our knowledge: 'It is clear that the tools for the recognition of previous brain damage are grossly inadequate and that the cause for behavioural aberrations in many instances must go undiscovered.'

There is general agreement, at the phenomenological level, about the interaction of a variety of malfunction covering, to quote from Birch's summary,[5] developmental lag, behaviour disturbance, motor awkwardness, minor perceptual disturbance, distractibility. He might have added a number of symptoms indicative of inefficient neural control or regulation of the soma – poor vocal articulation, faults of homeostasis, enuresis, excessive sweating or salivation, choroid movements, restless or over-heavy sleep, 'hysterical' pains and disabilities. What is uncertain is the nature of the morphological or metabolic counterparts of these phenomena. Birch points out that a diagnosis of brain damage, even if qualified as diffuse or minimal, is presumptive in the absence of evidence of actual damage to the cerebral structure. Yet 'brain damage' has acquired currency as a term covering this field of knowledge. Birch retains the term, but insists that it 'refers to a behaviour syndrome and not to the fact of brain damage as such'. One might question whether it would not be better to drop a misleading description in favour of a less tendentious one such as neural impairment or neural dysfunction.

APPENDIX I

The Delinquency Prediction Instrument

The preliminary sorting procedure of the Delinquency Prediction Instrument consists of six questions, as below, in answer to which the teacher marks Yes or No:

1. Is he a nuisance, or does he take correction badly? Yes/No
2. Has he been involved in wanton damage to property, truancy, or dishonest or other undesirable behaviour? Yes/No
3. Does he choose as companions children who might lead him into such? Yes/No
4. Is he untrustworthy, or sly, so that it is hard to 'pin anything on him'? Yes/No
5. Is he apt to be on bad terms with other children, or make himself disliked by bullying, spitefulness, or underhand tricks? Yes/No
6. Does he play to the gallery, show off, boast, or let himself be dared into foolish pranks? Yes/No

The figures below summarize the incidence of unfavourable answers in respect of boys and girls in ten of the twelve schools that formed the basis of the investigation reported in Part I. It will be remembered that the children who were assessed were in the twelve to thirteen year-group. They are not a representative sample since all the schools were situated in high-delinquency areas.

It is seen that, as would be anticipated, girls showed fewer of the types of behaviour associated with delinquency in comparison with

Incidence of unfavourable answers.

	No. of questions answered unfavourably						
	0	*1*	*2*	*3*	*4*	*5*	*6*
560 boys	360	66	57	31	25	15	6
%	*64·3*	*11·8*	*10·2*	*5·5*	*4·5*	*2·7*	*1·1*
474 girls	367	51	24	12	8	6	6
%	*77·6*	*10·8*	*5·1*	*2·5*	*1·7*	*1·3*	*1·3*

boys. But the difference between the sexes was even greater in respect of the number of actual offences that were committed. These findings suggest, first, that girls are somewhat less liable than boys to behaviour disturbance and, second, that, in girls, disturbance tends to take forms that less often lead to delinquency.

It is also noteworthy, in view of theories that delinquent and allied behaviour is part of the normal pattern of growing up in a delinquent neighbourhood, that nearly two-thirds of the boys and three-quarters of the girls exhibited no type of delinquency-associated behaviour.

The Delinquency Prediction Instrument itself is based upon those items in the Bristol Social Adjustment Guides found to be most closely associated with delinquency. The items are weighted according to the degree of this association as found in the Glasgow probation survey.[64, 65] The provisional norms thus established and the estimated chance of delinquency for each score-group are included in the general manual to the Bristol Social Adjustment Guides.[76]

APPENDIX II

Family Patterns and Types of Maladjustment

Family Patterns

The twelve patterns of family situation that have been found to be conducive to maladjustment or delinquency are summarized below:

Pattern A

Severe parental quarrelling, with the mother threatening to desert, or even doing so for short periods. The child is likely to show mother-anxiety symptoms (wanting to do her housework for her, buying her presents, giving her more than would be expected from his earnings); or, alternatively, avoidance symptoms (never in the house, frequenting amusement arcades, etc.). Often there will be hostility to the mother (if the child sees her as likely to abandon the family), and possibly a fantasy idealization of the father. Usually the child refuses to admit any family trouble, vaguely declaring that he is happy at home. He is usually of the XA/HA type.

Pattern B

Deep estrangement between the parents, although they are still living together. The mother attempts to satisfy her thwarted need for affection by over-indulging her son, especially the eldest, and using him as a means of spiting her husband. A violent antagonism grows up between father and son, with the son openly blaming the father for the family troubles. The critical point is reached when the mother's nerves break under the strain and she also turns on the boy, accusing him of being the source of the trouble. He is usually of the HA/K type.

More rarely, a reverse Pattern B is found, with the father emphasizing his estrangement from his wife by favouring a child.

Pattern C

The slum-breakdown family, the central feature of which is that the mother has 'given up', no longer making any effort to keep the house clean or to provide regular meals, becoming quite unconcerned about civilized standards, and leading an animal-like hand-to-mouth existence. This is due more often to depression than to mental subnormality, and there will almost certainly be weaknesses and stresses characteristic of the other patterns: parental quarrelling, mental and physical ill health in the father. The child is likely to be made anxious by threats of the mother to desert or to take her own life, and will suffer gross physical neglect and possibly ill treatment. This state of affairs should be distinguished from the low living standards of the happy-go-lucky family who are 'getting along', however dirty and untidy their home may be.

Pattern D

Characterized by mental ill health in the mother, with the father not sufficiently available as an alternative source of interest and security. The criterion is that the mother's mental disturbance has reached a stage where the strain of living with her has become almost unbearable, and her husband has taken the easy way out of finding a type of job, or a part-time recreation or interest that results in his being seldom in the house.

Pattern E

Its basis is a failure of maternal concern for the child, often resulting in the child's being left to a grandmother or other woman to bring up. Consequently the child will make his primary affectional attachments with the mother surrogate or with the father. So long as the child has the alternative source of security, breakdown will be unlikely, but a crisis may occur if it fails owing to death, desertion, or removal to another neighbourhood. This pattern, and Pattern I below, give rise to the state of conflict in the child named divided maternal attachment.

Pattern F

The emotional rejection of the child by the father. This may be due to his being away during the child's early years, or to early (possibly congenital) disturbance in the child which the father interprets as 'badness'. The pattern becomes critical when the father comes to regard the child as the traditional 'black sheep', fears that the other children will become infected with his naughtiness, and decides to 'cut his losses' in respect of the rejected child. The situation often causes quarrels between the parents, which may be resolved by the mother's also turning against the child for the sake of the family peace. The threats to have the child put away produce the counter-reaction of self-banishing hostility: the child resorts to provocative nuisance with the unconscious purpose of getting himself more decisively rejected. The result is a vicious circle of more drastic threats of putting away, and more nuisance, running away, and stealing within the home. Often the situation is provoked by the anxious-hostile personality of the father, but it can also arise with high-principled parents who take too serious a view of childish lying and other naughtiness. The child is usually of the XA/HA type.

Pattern G

Its origin is in the father's throwing undue strains on the mother, by his sickness and inability to work, by his unbalanced behaviour, or by his lack of support in running the family. The combination of mental stresses, sheer physical overwork, and inability to manage her family may induce in the mother a state of irritable-depressive non-tolerance, so that she reacts violently against any source of disturbance or annoyance. She may even temporarily express a vehement dislike of her child and demand that he be taken off her hands. A similar reaction is sometimes seen in mothers who have lost the support of their husbands by death or desertion.

Pattern H

Parental indifference and neglect. This pattern is comparatively rare, despite popular attribution of delinquency to a vague deficiency of parental affection. It is characterized by the parents' continually leaving their young family to fend for themselves while they pursue their evening's or weekend's pleasures. It should not be confused with the myth of the 'latch-key kid'. Children whose mothers go out to work have proved to be slightly less delinquent than those of stay-at-home mothers.

Pattern I

Its theme is the child's preference from his early years for some adult other than a parent. This is usually a grandmother who, by her spoiling and shielding of the child against the mother's discipline, has come to be regarded as the source of kindness and of all good things, while the mother is rejected as the one who denies and punishes. With the disappearance of the grandmother or other mother-figure the child cannot easily reverse the attitudes he has developed towards the true mother. The latter may in turn be unable to exercise any discipline, and allows herself to be imposed upon because of her anxiety about gaining her child's affection. The child is also subject to deep-seated anxiety because he cannot feel accepted by a mother who has been spurned. This form of divided maternal attachment is essentially one of conflict between looking to the mother-figure of the early years, who is ceasing to be an effective one, and being unable to reverse an attitude of rejection against the available true mother. It often happens, on the other hand, that a mother and grandmother can share amicably in the bringing up of a child, just as two parents can, without giving rise to emotional conflicts.

Pattern J

Centres on the child's fear of abandonment, often arising from a feature of the situation rather than from lack of parental affection. Instances are when the parents toy with the offer of a childless couple in better circumstances to adopt the child, and the state of uncertainty as to what will happen to the children in a pending divorce. A widowed mother may produce the same anxieties if she becomes so preoccupied with a new courtship that the child feels he will be forgotten in the event of her remarrying. The mother of an illegitimate child may make constant efforts to get him placed in an institution or foster-home because he is an embarrassment to her in her employment. A foster-mother who has had a child for many years and has become the effective mother may not feel that she has a right to resist the demand of the true mother, who may be a stranger to the child, to have him back. The fear of abandonment in such cases may induce in the child an inhibition of the capacity to make affectional attachments, together with violent hostility.

Pattern K

The parent to whom the child looks for affection gives the appearance of yielding to pressure to have him removed from the family. The most common situation in which this occurs is where there is an antagonistic step-parent. (But step-parent situations are not always of this sort: most provide the child with a sense of stability; in others the child actually looks to the step-parent for the stability and affection which the true parent is not giving, and the breakdown may occur following disappointment.) An elder sibling or grand-parent living in the home may also become antagonistic to the child and be constantly on at the parent to have the child removed because of his nuisance.

Pattern L

Arises from the anxiety of the child about losing the effective parent owing to ill health, old age, or threats of suicide. Where there is a second parent to fall back on this anxiety is unlikely to cause break-down. It is a principle of diagnosis that the presence of one reliable parent meets the child's needs for permanency in his family attachment.

Types of Maladjustment

Chapter Nine gave some account of the writer's approach to the problem of classifying disturbed behaviour. The various types of maladjustment that have been identified are designated by code letters on the Bristol Social Adjustment Guides, for purposes of diagnosis and scoring. For the reader's convenience, the code letters referred to in this volume are listed below, together with a brief description of the type of maladjustment that they represent.

U Unforthcomingness: inhibited lack of confidence before any difficulty or new situation; a defect of natural assertiveness and curiosity, usually congenital.

D Depression: from ups and downs of energy and irritability to continuous depression and neuro-physical exhaustion.

W Withdrawal: the child sets up defences against human contact and against being loved.

K An attitude of unconcern for adult approval and a 'writing off' of adults; ranging from a lack of desire to please and a lack of fellow-feeling and compunction in minor matters to a serious loss of human feeling and moral impairment.

XA Anxiety or uncertainty about adult interest and affection; includes seeking attention and being over-demanding of affection, and great anxiety for acceptance.

HA Hostility to adults: from a mildly rejecting attitude to active hostility showing itself in antisocial behaviour; in its most serious form, uncontrolled habitual hostility.

HC Hostility to other children: from jealous rivalry to enmity and lack of human feeling.

XC Anxiety for approval of and acceptance by other children, sometimes to the extent of being led into mischief.

R Restlessness: an inability to persevere, concentrate, or reflect, and a liking for easy moment-to-moment satisfactions – the avoidance response to acute anxiety or a congenital disorganization of motivation and behaviour.

See pp. 169–72 above for discussion of the more recently formulated inconsequential syndrome, which comprises aspects of R, XC, and XA.

APPENDIX III

Three Examples of Borderline Maladjustment

In a number of studies in which the Bristol Social Adjustment Guides[76] have been used as a means of measuring behaviour disturbance, the criterion of 20 indications has been chosen as the statistical borderline of maladjustment. The incidence of maladjustment as thus defined (see Chapter Six) may appear rather high. In order that the reader can judge what this criterion means in real terms three children at or near the borderline score have been picked from the sample of truants and their controls described in Chapter Seven. Their cases illustrate some of the commonest types of behaviour disturbance.

1. Boy, aged 11 years, non-truant, showing hostility with some depression and inconsequence

Total score 20 (9HA; 2K; 5D; 2XC; 1R; 1M)

BSAG category	*Items marked by teacher*
Greeting teacher	sometimes eager, sometimes definitely avoids
Helping teacher with jobs	offers except when in bad mood
Answering questions	eager except when in one of his moods
General manner with teacher	sometimes friendly, sometimes in a bad mood
Talking to teacher	inclined to be moody
Truthfulness	sometimes a fluent liar
Attitude to correction	resentful muttering or expression at times
Effect of correction	bears a grudge; always regards punishment as unfair
Ability at class jobs	varies with moods

BSAG category	*Items marked by teacher*
Contacts with teacher	minimizes contacts, but not backward with other children
Attentiveness	won't bother to learn
Asking teacher's help	depends on how he feels
Persistence (class work)	can work alone but has no energy
Persistence (manual tasks)	impatient; loses temper with job
Eyes	dull, listless
Posture	slumps, lolls about
Liking the limelight	misbehaves when teacher is out of the room
Nuisance	foolish pranks when with a gang
Belongings	careless, untidy; often loses or forgets books, pen
Punctuality	often late

2. Boy, aged 14 years, truant, showing high K (rejection of adults)

Total score 21 (10K; 4D; 2W; 2R; 2M)

BSAG category	*Items marked by teacher*
Helping teacher with jobs	has no wish to volunteer
Answering questions	not shy but unconcerned
Asking teacher's help	not shy but never comes for help willingly
General manner with teacher	not open or friendly
Talking to teacher	avoids teacher but talks to other children
Contacts with teacher	minimizes contacts but not backward with other children
Effect of correction	treats lenience as weakness
Persistence (classwork)	only works when watched or compelled
Eyes	can't look you in the face
Liking for attention	unconcerned about approval or disapproval
Asking teacher's help	too apathetic to bother
Classroom behaviour	has no life in him
Attentiveness	apathetic ('just sits')
Posture	slumps, lolls about
Greeting teacher	absolutely never greets
Companionship	distant
Standard (manual)	rough and ready, slapdash
Belongings	careless, untidy
Attitude of other children	on the fringe, somewhat of an outsider
Attendance	has truanted once or twice

3. Girl, aged 12 years, non-truant, showing severe unforthcomingness

Total score 20 (11U; 1W; 5D; 1K; 2M)

BSAG category	*Items marked by teacher*
Greeting teacher	waits to be noticed before greeting
Response to greeting	mumbles shyly, awkwardly
Helping teacher with job	never offers but pleased if asked
Answering questions	gets nervous, blushes
Asking teacher's help	too shy to ask
Talking to teacher	says very little; never makes any first approach
Liking for sympathy	likes sympathy but reluctant to ask
Team games	submissive, takes less wanted position
Informal play	shrinks from active play
Companionship	associates only with one other child and mostly ignores the rest
Attentiveness	dreamy
Persistence (manual tasks)	lacks physical energy
Team games	always sluggish, lethargic
Speech	inaudible
Eyes	listless
Expression	seldom smiles
Contacts with teacher	minimizes contacts but not backward with other children
Team games	timid; can't let herself go
Fidgets, etc.	makes aimless movements with hands

APPENDIX IV

Techniques of Diagnosis

In dealing with the situation of a child within his family the caseworker is faced with a bewildering array of observations. The variables are in effect so subtle and complex that many workers are induced to proclaim that 'every case is unique'. If this were absolutely true there would be no possibility of gaining any knowledge or understanding, for there would be no regularities to act as a guide to insight.

We apparently have instinctive means for appraising human attitudes, and these often stand the caseworker or teacher who is acting in a counselling capacity in good stead. Naturally, also, the sensitive caseworker will intuitively generalize from experience, and a number of standard causes of tension are thereby recognized. But without explicit theory and techniques of diagnosis insight is unreliable, and we are at the mercy of fashionable but unauthenticated conceptions. These are given a certain plausibility in that they seem to tally with observation, but the direction of cause and effect is apt to be taken for granted. A mother thought to be mollycoddling an extremely confidence-lacking child is accused of overprotection and urged to let him 'stand on his own feet'; in effect he may have suffered a congenital impairment of confidence which has been recognized by an affectionate mother. Many mothers are held responsible for the child's maladjustment because they are found in a rejecting mood; the truth may be that their children were always difficult and unrewarding in a way that would have induced rejection in a normally affectionate mother once her tolerance threshold had been overstepped.

Apart from our professional misconceptions we are dealing with a field of knowledge which was formerly the preserve of popular lore and one in which many non-specialists claim to know the answers. As a member of a particular cultural grouping the family caseworker will be under the influence of traditions and anti-traditions, each according to his or her individual temperament or upbringing. Our knowledge, as is evident from the present study, is also at the formative stage. In such a situation diagnosis and the formulation of a treatment plan are best subjected to the checks of a case conference.

The main drawback to this procedure is the time that is liable to be taken up with the circumstantial reporting of each case. If the conference is going to cover a worthwhile number of cases some kind of limitation to the discussion has to be agreed upon. Much time is often wasted in exploring the reasons for the mother's supposed affectional inadequacies, which involves a recapitulation of the history of her own childhood as well as that of the child. Such information may be valuable if an intensive and prolonged course of therapy can be undertaken, but this is seldom possible with existing resources and the number of children needing help. Moreover, the status of this type of explanation is dubious, and if indulged in is likely to deflect the conference into theoretical controversy. Out of practical necessity it was agreed in the conferences at which the present cases were discussed to avoid speculation as to the *origin* of the parental personalities. Once one goes back to the parents' own childhoods there is no reason why one should not extend the inquiry to the personalities of the grandparents, and in turn to their childhoods.

It has to be clear what type of diagnosis is going to be of value. This is a matter of assessing two main variables: the degree of vulnerability of the child; and the nature of the stresses to which he is, and has been, subjected. Vulnerability can be assessed by study of the child's contemporary reactions in the home and school, corroborated by evidence of somatic-neural impairment and any history of early dysfunction and/or trauma. The latter should ideally include prenatal and birth complications. The stressfulness of the child's family situation is chiefly a matter of assessing, from objective indications, the attitudes of the parents or surrogate parent towards the child as they then are, and an attempt to understand how deleterious attitudes have developed. From the point of view of treatment it is important to decide how far these may be the result of special stresses to which the parent has been subjected (deriving from economic vicissitudes, the other marriage partner, the child himself, another child, ill health, etc.) or are ingrained in the parent's personality. Such insight may emerge only in the course of family therapy, and in any case the initial diagnosis will need operational confirmation. The assessment of the nature of the stress and the degree to which it may be alleviated is thus centred upon contemporary, concrete observations.

The application of these diagnostic principles demands the use of systematic techniques and instruments. A freely written report, besides being a burdensome and time-consuming chore for which few caseworkers have any liking, is usually unstructured, unwieldy, and full of gaps. It was rendered unnecessary in the present conferences by the use of the Child-in-the-Family schedule of the Bristol Social Adjustment Guides and the inset Life-History Chart. Instead of laboriously composing a report upon a home visit, the caseworker has merely to underline on the schedule a number of alternative phrases. Where a particular piece of information is not provided for, a marginal annotation can be made. In this way no essential factor is easily overlooked, and any other person who is experienced in the use of the schedule can quickly make an appraisal of the family situation by a rapid scanning of the underlined phrases and annotations. For those without such special experience the observations should be entered in the appropriate spaces of the Diagnostic Form, and their import summarized in terms of parent-child attitudes. The value of this type of structured, systematic reporting procedure is often seen by the bringing to light of, for example, the influence of an adult other than the parent, which a caseworker could otherwise forget to inquire about. The child's history – the adults with whom he has lived from birth, changes of parent figures, illnesses, separations, onset of behaviour disturbances, stability of siblings, etc. – can similarly be entered graphically and by annotation without recourse to free composition. The method enables the story of the child's development to be visually grasped in a minute or two. In the case conferences a tentative diagnosis could be arrived at by the use of these instruments within a few minutes. This would be corroborated or corrected by the further information which the caseworker could give from first-hand experience. Where supplementary information was needed for corroboration or in order to decide between alternative diagnostic possibilities, the caseworker knew what to look for or inquire about on revisit. The time taken for the first comprehensive review of a case and the formulation of the first steps of a treatment plan averaged no more than half an hour.

Bibliography

1. ADAMSON, J. (1960), *Born Free*. Glasgow: Collins.

2. ADER, R. & BELFER, M. L. (1962). Prenatal maternal anxiety and offspring emotionality in the rat. *Psychol. Rep.* **10,** 711–18.

3. AINSWORTH, M. D. (1962). The effects of maternal deprivation: a review of findings and controversy in the context of research strategy. In *Deprivation of maternal care*, pp. 97–165. Geneva: World Health Organization.

4. ASUNI, T. (1963). Acculturation problems arising in Africa. *International Mental Health Newsletter* **5,** 11.

5. BIRCH, H. G. (ed.) (1964). *Brain damage in children: its biological and social aspects.* Baltimore: Williams and Wilkins.

6. BOWLBY, J., AINSWORTH, M. D., BOSTON, M. & ROSENBLUTH, D. (1956). The effects of mother–child separation: a follow-up study. *Brit. J. med. Psychol.* **29,** 211–47.

7. BURTON, L. (1964). Three studies of deviant child development. Ph.D. thesis, Queen's University, Belfast.

8. CASLER, L. (1961). Maternal deprivation: a critical review of the literature. *Mon. Soc. Res. Child Devel. No. 80,* **26,** No. 2.

9. CHAZAN, M. (1963). Maladjustment, attainment and sociometric status. *Collegiate Faculty of Education Journal,* Swansea.

10. CLEGG, A. B. (1961). Caning, behaviour and delinquency in secondary schools. West Riding County Council Education Committee, Wakefield, Yorks.

11. CLEGG, A. B. (1962). The role of the school. In *Delinquency and discipline*. London: Councils and Education Press.

12. COMMAND PAPER 2051 (1963). Statistics relating to approved schools, remand homes and attendance centres in England and Wales for the year 1961. London: HMSO.

13. CUNNISON, J. & GILFILLAN, J. B. S. (1951). Third Statistical Account of Scotland. Glasgow: Collins.

14. DOUGLAS, J. W. B. & MULLIGAN, D. G. (1961). Emotional adjustment and educational achievement. *Proc. roy. Soc. Med.* **54,** 885–91.

15. DRILLIEN, C. M. (1964). *The growth and development of the prematurely born infant.* Edinburgh: Livingstone.

16. FERGUSON, T. (1962). *The young delinquent in his social setting.* London: Oxford University Press.

17. FRASER, F. CLARKE, KALTER, H., WALKER, B. E. & FAINSTAT, T. D. (1954). Experimental production of cleft palate with cortisone and other hormones. *J. cellular compar. Physiol.* **43,** Suppl. 1, 237–59.

18. FRENCH, M. P. (1958). Personality traits and the moral insight of the young vandals. Bachelor of Education thesis, Glasgow University.

19. GILES, G. (1959). The validation of the Bristol Social Adjustment Guide for Glasgow children. Bachelor of Education thesis, Glasgow University.

20. GLUECK, S. & E. (1950). *Unraveling juvenile delinquency.* New York: Commonwealth Fund.

21. GOLDFARB, W. (1943–4). Effects of early institutional care on adolescent personality. *J. experimental Educ.* **12,** 106–29.

22. GOLDFARB, W. (1945–6). Effects of psychological deprivation in infancy and subsequent stimulation. *Amer. J. Psychiat.* **102,** 18–33.

23. GÖLLNITZ, G. (1954). *Die Bedeutung der frühkindlichen Hirnschädigung für die Kinderpsychiatrie.* Leipzig: Thieme.

24. GÖLLNITZ, G. (1961). Über die Milieuänfalligkeit des Hirngeschädigten Kindes. In H. Schwarz, *Das milieugeschädigte Kind.* Jena: Fischer.

25. GÖLLNITZ, G. (1963–4) Über die Problematik der Neurosen im Kindesalter. *Ideggyogyaszati Szemle,* 97–108.

26. HARLOW, H. F. (1962). Development of affection in primates. In E. L. Bliss (ed.), *Roots of behavior.* New York: Harper.

27. HEARNSHAW, L. S. (1956). Temporal integration and behaviour. *Bull. Brit. psychol. Soc.* **30,** 1–20.

28. HUMPHREY, M. E. & ZANGWILL, O. L. (1951). Cessation of dreaming after brain injury. *J. Neurol. Neurosurg. Psychiat.* **14,** 322–5.

29. INGRAM, T. T. S. (1956). A characteristic form of overactive behaviour in brain-damaged children. *J. ment. Sci.* **102,** 550–8.

30. JEPHCOTT, A. P. & CARTER, M. P. (1954). *The social background of delinquency.* Nottingham University.

31. JUNG, C. G. (1924). *Pyschological types.* London: Kegan Paul.

32. KARN, M. N. & PENROSE, L. S. (1961). Birth weight and gestation time in relation to maternal age, parity and infant survival. *Ann. Eugenics* **16,** 147–64.

33. KEELEY, K. (1962). Prenatal influence on behaviour of offspring of crowded mice. *Science* **135,** 44–5.

34. KÖHLER, W. (1924). *The mentality of apes.* London: Routledge & Kegan Paul.

35. LEWIS, H. (1954). *Deprived children.* London: Nuffield Foundation and Oxford University Press.

36. LORENZ, K. (1959). *Man meets dog.* London: Methuen and Pan Books.

37. MALPAS, P. (1937) The incidence of human malformations and the significance of changes in the maternal environment in their causation. *J. Obstet. Gynaecol. Brit. Emp.* **44,** 434–54.

38. MANSON, M. N., LOGAN, W. P. D. & LOY, R. M. (1960). Rubella and other virus infections during pregnancy. *Ministry of Health Reports No. 101.* London.

38a. MARSHALL, A. G., HUTCHINSON, E. O. & HONISETT, J. (1962). Heredity in common diseases: a retrospective study of twins in a hospital population. *Brit. med. J.,* January, pp. 1–6.

39. MAYS, J. B. (1962). *Education and the urban child.* Liverpool: Liverpool University Press.

40. MAYS, J. B. (1962). The influence of environment. In *Delinquency and discipline.* London: Councils and Education Press.

41. MAYS, J. B. (1963). Delinquency areas – a reassessment. *Brit. J. Criminol.* **3**, 216–30.

42. MCCORD, W. & MCCORD, J. (1959). *Origins of crime.* New York: Columbia University Press.

43. NISSEN, H. W. (1954). The nature of the drive as innate determinant of behavioural organization. In M. R. Jones (ed.), *Nebraska Symposium on motivation*, pp. 281–321. Lincoln: Nebraska University Press.

44. O'CONNOR, N. (1956). Evidence for the permanently disturbing effects of mother–child relationships. *Acta Psychologica* **12**, 174.

45. PENFIELD, W. (1954). Studies of the cerebral cortex of man. A review and an interpretation. In J. F. Delafresnaye (ed.), *Brain mechanisms and consciousness.* Oxford: Blackwell.

46. PRECHTL, H. F. R. (1961). Neurological sequelae of pre-natal and para-natal complications. In B. M. Foss (ed.), *Determinants of infant behaviour*, pp. 45–8. London: Methuen; New York: Wiley.

47. PRECHTL, H. F. R. & STEMMER, CH. J. (1962). The choreiform syndrome in children. *Devel. Med. Child Neurol.* **4**, 119–27.

48. PROCTER, M. (1958). Tutorial classes. *Education Bulletin No. 445.* London County Council.

49. ROPER, W. E. (1950, 1951). A comparative study of the Wakefield Prison population in 1948 and 1949. *Brit. J. Delinq.* **1**, Nos. 1 and 4.

50. SCHAFFER, H. R. (1958). Objective observations of personality development in early infancy. *Brit. J. med. Psychol.* **31**, 174–83.

51. SCHAFFER, H. R. & EMERSON, P. E. (1964). The development of social attachments in infancy. *Mon. Soc. Res. Child Devel.* **29**, iii. No. 94.

52. SEILER, H. E. (1957). Annual report of the Public Health Department, Edinburgh (quoted by Drillien).

53. SMITH, MORRISON J. (1961). Prevalence and natural history of asthma in schoolchildren. *Brit. med. J.* i, 711–13.

54. SPINLEY, B. M. (1953). *The deprived and the privileged.* London: Routledge.

55. STOTT, D. H. (1950). *Delinquency and human nature.* Dunfermline, Fife: Carnegie United Kingdom Trust.

56. STOTT, D. H. (1956). *Unsettled children and their families.* London: University of London Press; New York: Philosophical Library.

57. STOTT, D. H. (1957). Physical and mental handicaps following a disturbed pregnancy. *Lancet* i, 18 May, 1006–12.

58. STOTT, D. H. (1959). Some psychosomatic aspects of casualty in reproduction. *J. psychosom. Res.* **3**, 42–55.

59. STOTT, D. H. (1959). Evidence for pre-natal impairment of temperament in mentally retarded children. *Vita Humana* **2**, 125–48.

60. STOTT, D. H. (1959). Infantile illness and subsequent mental and emotional development. *J. genet. Psychol.* **94**, 233–51.

61. STOTT, D. H. (1960). Delinquency, maladjustment and unfavourable ecology. *Brit. J. Psychol.* **51**, 157–70.

62. STOTT, D. H. (1960). Observation on retest discrepancy in mentally subnormal children. *Brit. J. educ. Psychol.* **30,** 211–19.

63. STOTT, D. H. (1960). Interaction of heredity and environment in regard to 'measured intelligence'. *Brit. J. educ. Psychol.* **30,** 95–102.

64. STOTT, D. H. (1960). The prediction of delinquency from non-delinquent behaviour. *Brit. J. Delinq.* **10,** 195–210.

65. STOTT, D. H. (1960). A new delinquency prediction instrument using behavioural indications. *Internat. J. soc. Psychiat.* **5,** 195–205.

66. STOTT, D. H. (1961). An emprical approach to motivation based on the behaviour of a young child. *J. Child Psychol. Psychiat.* **2,** 97–117.

67. STOTT, D. H. (1962). Evidence for a congenital factor in maladjustment and delinquency. *Amer. J. Psychiat.* **118,** 781–94.

68. STOTT, D. H. (1962). Delinquency and cultural stress. *Brit. J. soc. clin. Psychol.* **1,** 182–91.

69. STOTT, D. H. (1962). Cultural and natural checks to population growth. In M. F. A. Montagu (ed.), *Culture and the evolution of man.* New York: Oxford University Press.

70. STOTT, D. H. (1962). Abnormal mothering as a cause of mental subnormality, Part I. *J. Child Psychol. Psychiat.* **3,** 79–91.

71. STOTT, D. H. (1962). Abnormal mothering as a cause of mental subnormality, Part II. *J. Child Psychol. Psychiat.* **3.** 133–48.

72. STOTT, D. H. (1963). Delinquency proneness and court disposal of young offenders. *Brit. J. Criminol.* **4,** 37–42.

73. STOTT, D. H. (1964). Sociological and psychological explanations of delinquency. *Internat. J. soc. Psychiat.* Special Congress Number.

74. STOTT, D. H. (1965). Family-situations conducive to behaviour-disturbance in a delinquent group. *Social Work* **10,** ii, 14–17.

75. STOTT, D. H. (1965). *The social adjustment of children.* Manual to the Bristol Social Adjustment Guides. Including the Delinquency Prediction Instrument. 3rd edn. London: University of London Press.

76. STOTT, D. H. & SYKES, E. G. (1956). *The Bristol Social Adjustment Guides.* London: University of London Press.

77. SYMONDS, C. (1962). Concussion and its sequelae. *Lancet* i, 1–5.

78. THOMPSON, W. R. (1957). Influence of prenatal maternal anxiety on emotionality in young rats. *Science* **125,** 698–9.

79. WILSON, H. (1962). *Delinquency and child neglect.* London: Allen & Unwin.

80. WYNNE-EDWARDS, V. E. (1962). *Animal dispersion in relation to social behaviour.* Edinburgh: Oliver and Boyd.

81. YARROW, L. J. (1961). Maternal deprivation: toward an empirical and conceptual re-evaluation. *Psychol. Bull.* **58,** 459–90.

82. YOUNG, M. & WILLMOTT, P. (1956). *Family and kinship in East London.* London: Routledge.

Index

For Product Safety Concerns and Information please contact our EU representative GPSR@taylorandfrancis.com Taylor & Francis Verlag GmbH, Kaufingerstraße 24, 80331 München, Germany